FATAL WORDS FRAGILE HOPES

Mental Disorders in Children Traumas and Treatments

Seaon Ducote

Marina Sharfman

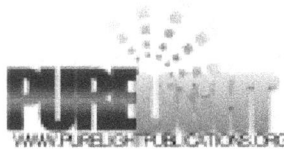

Purelight Publications
Dallas Texas
http://www.purelightpublications.org

Library of Congress Cataloging-in Publications Data
Ducote, Billie Seaon
Fatal Words Fragile Hopes/
Mental Disorders in Children/Traumas and Treatments

ISBN 9780615234328
ISBN 0615234321

Printed in the United States
Cover Illustration & Design
by Seaon Ducote

Edited by Purelight Publications
Sydney Kunz-McCarthy

Printed in the United States of America
First Printing

Dedicated

to

new

beginnings...

Acknowledgment

**We wish to thank the doctors who have contributed to this book,
and for the personal sacrifices they have made in their life
to bring to light the true and natural art of healing.**

Einstein is thought to have struggled with autism
as a child (unable to speak until he was 3 years of age.
His school years were a struggle, often needing the help
of classmates to do, or help with homework. As a college
student he was marginalized by his professors as a dreamer,
a "C student," scorned by fellow scientists as an oddity, yet
his Theory of Relativity changed the world, bringing forth
THE NUCLEAR AGE.

Any one of the many levels of obsessive compulsion manifested by the creative mind, can reach genius proportions, often applauded, envied and revered by the world. But only friends and family are familiar with the agony that is experienced with this need to achieve works of amazing proportions.

And when it happens that they break the barrier of normalcy, we stand in awe of the beauty and knowledge they have achieved, knowing in our heart that such works could only have been captured by their obsessive compulsion to manifest that need.

Seaon Ducote

CONTENTS

FATAL WORDS FRAGILE HOPES

TRAUMAS

Mental Disorders In Children

The Quest For Answers
Seaon Ducote

The tests were finished. The results, neatly typed, now lay in-wait for the doctor's review. It was the moment of truth, a moment that the parents had long dreaded. They wanted their son back to normal, and had gone to great expense to find the answers that would heal their little boy. The father sat quietly, face drawn, arms tightly crossed, prepared for the worst. He glanced at his wife, sitting on the edge of her chair, smiling politely as she waited nervously to hear the doctor's plan. But the review quickly became a dark tunnel of endless words echoing through her mind, words leaving her in fear, with no hope for the future. The parents were shocked, tears stream down the mother's face as she sobbed, pleading for a solution. The doctor paused, removed his glasses and looked tenderly into the eyes of the parents.

"I'm sorry, but there simply is not a cure for Tourette Syndrome."

These words echo across the world each year, year after year. And year after year mothers and fathers weep for their children, branded with a spectrum of mental disorders labeled incurable. Each year they watch their children teetering on the edge, living moment to moment, waiting and dreading the senseless, unannounced parade of physical and mental forms of embarrassment. Because of the grief, and their own mental confusion, it is understandable that the majority believe their only hope for their child's peace of mind is to follow a series of mind-altering drug treatments offered by their family doctor.

On November 23, 2006, an article by Gardiner Harris, entitled, **"Proof Is Scant on Psychiatric Drug Mix for Young,"** was published in the New York Times. The following is an excerpt:

3

The F.D.A. requires drug makers to prove that their drugs work safely before the agency will approve them for sale in the United States. But doctors can prescribe and combine approved medicines as they see fit. Such mixing is common in medicine but rarely studied by drug makers.

"Psychiatrists started mixing psychiatric medications because the drugs were only moderately effective and often caused terrible side effects," said Dr. Steven E. Hyman, the provost of Harvard University and former director of the National Institute of Mental Health. "None of these drugs by themselves do an adequate job of controlling symptoms," Dr. Hyman said.

But in today's society it is no longer a secret with homeopathic practitioners, and many medical doctors that mental disorders in children can be safely treated with alternative medicine and supplements, in combination with cognitive therapy. Healthy treatments are therefore designed to include the attitudes and self-assessment of the parent' thoughts in helping to bring healing energy to the child.

Current research in neuroscience has inadvertently proven that the prophets, spiritual masters and Christian healers like Mary Baker Eddy and Charles Filmore were indeed correct in warning us that our body reacts according to positive or negative thoughts, via our fears, hopes, faith, hate and love. The current cutting edge brain imaging equipment enables research teams to view the blood flow to every area of the brain, measuring the brain's physical and emotional reactions to visual and audio input.

There is no doubt that our human brain reacts in its own unique pattern to every thought manifested in the brain, giving rise to the distinct possibility that the triggers of every mental disorder can someday be tracked and eventually healed. There is also another way to diagnose children with mental disorders. It is a simple and effective series of tests that few physicians offer or recommend to their patients.

Biomedical testing pinpoints the cause of metabolic disorders that can appear as mental and behavioral disorders, yet the majority of family physicians fail to order these tests before deciding to administer dangerous drugs to children. The reason usually revolves around the doctor's lack of knowledge of alternative methods. It is simply much easier to prescribe a mind altering drug. Therefore millions of children with mental disorders sit in Special Ed classes, embarrassed, feeling like they are inferior, because the majority of the medical profession still questions the proven and positive results of biomedical testing, alternative remedies and treatments.

The following is an example of what can happen without biomedical testing: According to the Mayo Clinic "Wilson's disease can cause abrupt personality changes and inappropriate behavior, that is often mis-diagnosed as behavioral problems because the child behaves erratically or performs poorly in school."

Wilson's disease is also associated with neurological signs and symptoms, such as tremors, muscle spasms, unsteady walk, difficulty speaking and drooling. So what is Wilson's disease? It is an accumulation of copper in the liver immediately after birth, but signs and symptoms rarely occur before the age of 5 or 6, and can also appear much later in life. It's time to ask ourselves why we are allowing children in America to go through the horrors of the side effects of drugs when the true culprits of their disorder could possibly be revealed through biomedical testing.

So, as we cross the threshold of a new era of healing, where spiritual and medical science are crossing paths, isn't it time to refrain from labeling any disorder or disease "incurable"? The words "incurable" and "terminal" have no business being thrust into the life of anyone fighting a mental or physical disorder or disease, especially when we are alerted daily of major medical and scientific advances. Many teens and adults branded "terminal" or "incurable" have taken their own lives when branded with death. And many others, through the prayers and positive words of hope from their friends and family, have proved doctors wrong by healing themselves.

I believe that we are perfect of mind, body and spirit, but our lifestyle and the negative actions and reactions we experience can literally breakdown our mind and body on a daily basis. Many adults have found it impossible to escape childhood without developing some form of self-destructive habit, mental disorder, disease, or family issues that lead to drug and alcohol addition. So, as a result, many children of these parents also walk through life with untreated depression, obsessive compulsive and bipolar disorders, abandonment issues, post traumatic stress, attention deficit hyperactivity, tics (Tourette Syndrome), and countless more disorders that physicians find more appropriate to remedy with psychotropic drugs, rather than pursue an alternative healing program. So, whom do we blame? Let's try blaming a healthcare system that America has long ago outgrown. We may wave our flags and hear the elegant speeches about equal opportunity, but there is no equal opportunity in America for those who cannot afford to pay for state of the art health care.

Our former First Lady Rosalynn Carter, founder of The Carter Center Mental Health Program, presents a positive outlook for children with mental disorders: "We know so much more about the brain and effective treatments than we did even a decade ago. There is mounting evidence that the trajectory of a child's life can be altered considerably in a positive way when treatment is provided early as possible." I have no doubt that she is correct, provided that the parent has the funds and education to know where to take their child for the best treatments.

There is no doubt that neuroscience is on the cutting edge of revealinf brain malfunctions, but the fact is, if a solution for every mental disorder known today, became available tomorrow, our current 70 percent of children going untreated for lack of funds to hire the services of the very best in mental healthcare would continue until a change is made, not to reform, but to build a new healthcare system that also embraces treatment for mentally ill children currently incarcerated, in place of punishment.

Unfortunately, the family physician's treatment of mental disorders in children has rarely advanced beyond the practice of prescribing dangerous drugs. America is now seeing the result of that practice on many levels. On September 22, 2003, Bob Edwards, host of the Morning Show, introduced a report by NPR's Vicky Que, revealing that doctors were diagnosing an increasing number of younger aged children with serious mental disorders, and treating them with psychiatric drugs that had been developed for adults and had never been tested for use on children.

This problem is still very real, and is currently given as a warning in the opening statement on the Obsessive Compulsive Foundation website: **"Medication treatment should only be considered when children are experiencing significant OCD impairment or distress. Or when cognitive behavioral therapy is unavailable, or only partly effective."** **http://www.ocfoundation.org/ocd-medication-children.html**

The lack of treatment for mental disorders in children will continue to evolve into a mentally ill society with various levels of anger issues. Many social workers believe that this is exactly what we are facing in our society today because of the lack of free mental healthcare facilities. Current estimates of mentally ill children in the United States puts the number at 7 million **diagnosed cases**. This estimate does not include the 70 percent of children with mental disorders going without treatment. One can only imagine what social problems will arise from this neglect in our current and future generations.

According to **Human Rights Watch**, a federal statistics study in 2006 revealed that mentally ill inmates in U.S. prisons and jails had quadrupled over the past six years. More than half of all prison and state inmates now report mental health problems, including depression, mania and psychotic disorders, estimated to be 1.25 million.

The rate of reported mental health disorders in the state prison population is five times greater (56.2 percent) than in the general population (11 percent). These people are eventually released to deal with the stigma of their untreated mental disorders and the stigma of being an ex-con. Is it any wonder that our country has the highest prison population in the world?

The "bail-out legislation" of 2008 gave the mental healthcare a boost. *The New York Times* reported that more than one-third of all Americans will soon get better insurance coverage of mental health treatments because of a new law that requires equal coverage of mental and physical illnesses. But what about the remaining two-thirds of Americans who cannot afford healthcare insurance, or those who only receive basic healthcare through their employer?

On November 21, 2008, I sat watching a 20/20 documentary on Nebraska's Safe Haven Act. The law was put into effect to protect newborn babies being abandoned by unwed mothers. The Safe Haven Act allowed a parent to leave their child at any hospital, no questions asked. But, because law makers failed to insert age and state location limits into the Act, suddenly single mothers were driving from other states to leave their mentally ill children in Nebraska hospitals.

These were children with violent behavior, that neither the parent nor schools were able to control, nor provide with expensive neurological assessments. All of the mothers interviewed had at least one additional child at home that was being victimized by the violent sibling. Many of us were shocked. Were these bad mothers, giving away their children, or mothers victimized by a government unable to provide treatments and counseling, to those who cannot afford it?

This lack of lack of free mental healthcare is causing thousands of parents to turn to special diets and a variety of alternative treatments, including herbal remedies, for their children. Marina Sharfman is one of those parents. After eight years of watching her son go through a series of hellish side effects from numerous prescription drugs, and unable to get healthcare insurance, Marina and her husband took an alternative route for their son, suffering from a severe case of Tourette Syndrome, ADHD, OCD, and Bi-polar disorder.

A major portion of our healthcare system could be enhanced if the world of natural medicine were allowed to come forward in declaration of the truth about their success with natural treatments for children's mental disorders. Unfortunately, the AMA (American Medical Association) and the pharmaceutical companies have set forth the idea that biomedical tests and supplement treatments are not in the realm of legitimate healing practices. Many of us, however, know this way of thinking to be false. The fact is that all forms of healing methods should be voiced, studied and applied where appropriate to the situation, especially if a medical doctor has no treatment available other than psychotropic drugs.

In our society, ironically, spiritual and homeopathic healing still takes a back seat to drug products supplied by medical doctors. Healing mind and body with a combination of herbal and homeopathic remedies and prayer is still the last treatment that most parents seek; in fact, it would be wise to immediately incorporate prayer into beginning stages of any and all alternative or medical treatments. It is a scientific fact that individual and group prayer can heal disorders and diseases of all types, as you will discover in this book.

My own journey down the path of spiritual healing began when I was advised that I needed exploratory surgery to discover the cause of my protruding left eye. The day I was scheduled for surgery, the still small voice that speaks to me in times of trouble instructed me to run as fast as I could, to go home and wait for an answer. I quickly walked out of the hospital, prayed, and waited. The answer came about a week later, in the form of a referral by my husband's employer, to a Christian Science healer.

I was under such stress and depression when my husband suggested I visit her that I refused. I thought he had lost his mind. But after a couple of days of looking at my bulging eye in the mirror, I decided to go. I will never forget the day I walked into her office. Dorothy was a small woman with snow white hair and an aura around her that took my breath away. My visit was the first day of a 14 year student, teacher relationship. And yes, my eye was gradually healed over a 26 day period through a combination of her prayer work, and my re-affirming my oneness with God.

Over the years I began to understand that fear (a sort of unplugging from the God source) was the only thing that could separate me from my peace and oneness. It is truly a fact that when fear is vanquished from thought, the process of healing begins. This is especially true in helping children overcome physical and mental challenges.

Over the years I have witnessed many demonstrations of the power of prayer, especially in the protection and health it gave to my child. Soon after I began my metaphysics studies with my teacher/healer, I became pregnant. During my pregnancy I remained peaceful and creative. I made a commitment to learn the metaphysical reasons behind sickness and disease and to demonstrate it as far as my understanding would allow.

My baby daughter grew and blossomed over the years, shielded from all childhood vaccinations and popular explanations of what the medical world defined as sickness and disease. The result was a daughter, at the age of 18, who had never felt the pinch of a needle from any doctor, and never knew what it was like to have measles, chicken pox, or any other childhood disease. Her disposition sparkled as brightly as her perfect teeth when she left for college. Was my daughter perfect? No. At age 6 years of age she was fitted for glasses. But being perfect was not the point. As my teacher once reminded me, "If we were perfect, we would not be here." The point for me was to know and practice the truth of what a Human Being can be.

In the following pages you will follow the hardships surrounding Marina Sharfman and her son, Alex. Through the eight years of prescription drug horrors that Marina and her son experienced, she never stopped praying for an answer. Her story makes it clear that without her hope and daily prayers, I believe her son would have succumbed to one of the many tortures he experienced. There is no doubt that the prayers of a parent can turn the tide of any disorder.

I recently emailed a letter to President Obama, that detailed my thoughts on healthcare reform. My mother use to say that it was easier to make a new dress than to try and remake an old one. I envision healthcare as a ***human right*** in which men, women, and children from every walk of life are given the same quality of treatment. I hope for the formation of a system that accepts viable methods of healing from all spiritual, scientific, medical, and alternative practices of healing.

Alternative medicine, biomedical testing, supplements and homeopathic remedies and treatments are fast becoming the treatments of choice for those who are searching for healthy methods of healing not available through their family physicians. There can be no doubt that these methods have become the new and revised path to physical and mental health. Unfortunately, few insurance companies will cover alternative treatments, or biomedical testing.

So what do you do when you need something, but can't afford it? Well, as my grandmother use to say, "You best learn how to do it yourself. But before you start, you best ask God to show you the way."

Grandma was a wise ole soul and right on target with her advice. Many parents are applying this philosophy to alternative medicine, diet and supplements, as millions of Americans are taking matters into their own hands, tired of being refused treatment for lack of funds, or given shoddy, minimum care. Health food stores are booming with business because, believe it or not, it is not that difficult to learn how to take care of our children.

The Memoirs of Marina Sharfman

Dedicated to my husband.
You have encouraged me to write this experience for so long. Your words and images, along with your willingness to spend hours with me as I reached for clarity, have been critical to the evolution of this story. Thank you so much for helping me keep my sanity and patience throughout the years. I will love you forever. -Marina

Branded

We always knew that Alex was different from other children. At 2 years of age, Alex was angry, frustrated, and constantly crying. He acted out his frustration by throwing toys, or whatever he happen to be holding, at anyone who happened to walk into our home. There was no way that anyone could have mistaken his incessant crying and demanding for the normal actions of the "terrible twos." We had no idea that his inability to learn or to digest his surroundings was causing the frustration.

When Alex turned 3 years old, I signed registered him for a church program called "Mommy and Me." I was so excited. There were eighteen children and three teachers in his class. Our first week created a lot of frustration for Alex and the class. The crying began when Alex refused to participate according to the activity rules set up for the class. By the end of the second week his crying and behavior worsened, so I removed Alex from the program. He just couldn't grasp his place in the activities and interaction with the children.

I was heartbroken that my son seemed unable to have playmates, or understand simple instructions, so I decided to work with him at home. We started with ABCs. Eventually Alex was able to count to ten. Alex would receive an occasional birthday party invitation, allowing him to participate in free play (non-structured playtime) with children his age. They were special times for Alex and me. Little did I know how special they would come to be.

During Alex's third year I gave birth to my son, Dillon. I had a wonderful pregnancy and in many ways it was the highlight of Alex's life. Alex could not wait until his little brother was born. In the later months of my pregnancy with Dillon, Alex would touch my stomach to feel the baby kicking.

I was a little worried that Alex would be jealous of Dillon, because he was so attached to my husband and me, and our whole extended family. I began buying books to read to Alex that explained what it was like to have a new baby brother. I guess the books did the job; to my joy and surprise, Alex was never jealous of Dillon.

Alex would sit quietly, watching his grandfather hold Dillon in his arms, rocking his baby brother to sleep. Basically, Alex became a different child around his brother. Our demanding child became docile, loving and patient, expressing tenderness and love for his new brother. Over the years that love grew stronger, and to this day, they remain best friends.

The following year, as soon as Alex had his 4th birthday, we found a very impressive private pre-k school with three teachers to one class. They were amazing with Alex. To our amazement, Alex seemed to blossom that year. It was obvious that our high spirited child was going to grow out of his rebelliousness.

When Alex first entered kindergarten, there was no reason to believe that he would not, or could not, do the work. And as the year progressed we kept that belief, even when his teacher told us that she had to put Alex in "time-out" once or twice a day. The bottom line for me was that he was passing the grade and making friends.

Alex did pass on to the 1st grade, but my positive attitude about Alex's ability to be normal soon waned. He was slow and unable to comprehend instructions as simple as turning his book to a specific page. His teacher related that he always had a "lost look" on his face. Nevertheless, his lagging behind the other 23 children in the class didn't keep her from passing Alex to the 2nd grade. So, again, I rose to the occasion, believing that I could tutor Alex that summer, which would allow him to be prepared for the 2nd grade. I had done it once before and it helped, so I knew I could do it again.

Alex's behavior at home became worse than it had ever been. He was hyper and prone to temper tantrums, blinking his eyes and moving his head from side to side, then stopping for long periods of time, making it hard to discern what part of his behavior was intentional, anger oriented, or used to aggravate us. Little did we know, it was none of the above.

The 2nd grade was a repeat of the 1st grade. He demonstrated the same attention problems and inability to follow instructions; again, however, he was passed on to the 3rd grade. This time I made sure that he could keep pace with the class. I hired a tutor to work with him five days out of the week. She would review everything they covered in class and then help him study the assignments. Academically he began doing well, and seemed like a "normal" boy, Again, we were wrong.

Alex was on a neighborhood baseball team that year. We were proud of him; we knew it hard for our son to fit in with the kids. He tried, and we tried, to make things normal; but, inside we knew there was something we just couldn't fix. What it was, we didn't know, but watching him out on the field seemed to take the sting out of our lives for a brief time each week.

The end of our fantasy came quickly, exploding our lives into a million directions. It was a bright sunny day as Alex stepped up to the batter's box. He took on the usual batting stance, poised for the pitch, then suddenly it happened. Our son's head jerked to the side with such fury as to knock his helmet off of his head and onto the ground. My husband and I thought we were seeing things. Alex quickly leaned over, picked it up, and placed it back on his head, but, again, his head jerked so violently that the helmet was knocked to the ground.

I remember watching, as if it was a movie. It didn't seem real. I turned around to my sister-in-law, sitting on the bleacher behind us, to get her response. We weren't dreaming. She saw it too. We quickly put Alex in the car and headed for home. The movements progressed during the ride home, going from head jerking to constant clearing of his throat and incessant blinking. We had no idea what we were looking at; we just knew that our son was in trouble.

The following days were a nightmare. We immediately took Alex to see our pediatrician, and from there we were sent to a neurologist, who tested Alex with a complete brain scan. All he could tell us was that Alex had "tics" and needed a_complete neuropsychological evaluation. He referred us to a clinic in Long Island, New York. It was four months before they could give us an appointment, during which time the tics grew worse. Every day I watched my son fighting a battle with himself. He was pale; with dark circles under his beautiful blue eyes. He thought he was going crazy. He was crying, trying to stop the movements, but he was helpless.

It all seemed to be an endless cycle of days filled with worry and nights filled with tears. A constant stream of relatives came to visit Alex, some crying, some praying, all wondering when it would end. Finally, the evaluation day arrived.

The doctor explained the testing procedure, and what Alex would be doing over a three day period, six hours each day. A three day evaluation and ten days to get the results? The fear consumed me. Suddenly I knew that we were facing something that was not going away in one day.

Ten days later we sat in front of the doctor listening to him tell us that our son had Tourette Syndrome, associated with deficit/hyperactivity disorder, problems with organizational skills and working memory. I looked at the doctor in horror, wishing he would stop talking; but there was more: Alex also had a developmental language disorder, characterized by both expressive and receptive difficulty. I looked over at my husband. His face was as white as a ghost. We felt lost. We thought we would be getting solutions to Alex's problem; instead, we were told of more problems, none of which were presented with solutions.

I was angry and grief stricken. I heard the doctor say that he would be pleased to answer any questions. What questions? We were told that there was no cure for Tourette Syndrome, or ADHD, or any of his problems. NO CURE? It was the year 2000, and with all our technology, space ships, heart and organ transplants, cloning and a million other advances, we were told there was no help for our son.

My husband and I left the doctor's office, walked to our car, unlocked the door and burst into tears. We had lost a son to what? Names that meant nothing but a life of pain and embarrassment for Alex. We just sat there, going nowhere, holding each other as we drowned in a sea or sorrow.

When we arrived home we were faced with the next trauma. What would we tell Alex. He wanted to know what was wrong with him. My God! How could we explain something that even the doctors couldn't figure out. It's like telling someone that they are terminally ill, but will still live a long life.

We sat Alex down and explained to him in an honest, but delicate way that he had something called Tourette Syndrome and ADHD. The horror welled up in his eyes. He thought we were telling him that he was going to die. We quickly explained that it was not life-threatening and that he would live to be very old, but would have to take medicine to control the movements and sounds he was making.

Alex was relieved! However, he had no idea what T.S. was about. He was familiar with ADHD because some of his friends had it. But

Tourettes was something totally different. We told him it was a neurological disorder that he would most likely outgrow in his teen years. He asked what that meant and we told him that it meant that he had movements and sounds that he could not control. We were so afraid for our son's emotional state of mind. We didn't want him to think that we thought he was crazy or ill. We reminded him that he was a perfect child, even with the disorder called Tourette Syndrome.

Soon he grew very quiet and sad. No matter what we said to make him feel better he still felt sad; because now he saw himself as different from everyone around him. We tried to convince him otherwise, but to no avail. These conversations always ended with my husband and I holding Alex in our arms as he cried and cried, always assuring him that we would find the best doctors for him and keep trying to get the best help for him that we possibly could find.

Each time I watched him walk away, I couldn't help but wonder what was going on in my son's mind. Eventually our promise to find the best doctors, new research, and possible cures, came to an end when we were told that Alex could no longer get health care through any insurance company because of his mental disorders.

My husband and I finally decided to move to another state. We lived in a very upscale neighborhood, making life even harder for Alex. It was like living in the movie, "The Stepford Wives". The parents appeared to be perfect and nothing ever seemed to be wrong with their children. If there was a problem (which was rare), the child became isolated, and was no longer acknowledged by the neighbors. It would be the end of having playmates or invitations to birthday parties. And this was exactly what happened to Alex as soon as the news circulated that he had Tourette Syndrome.

It became apparent that we were left with only one solution. We had to find a location with a suitable neighborhood for our son. We sold our home that we had lived in for ten years. I think the worst part for all of us, especially Alex, was leaving our parents, aunts and uncles. Uncle Allen, Aunt Roseanne, Uncle Brian, Aunt Debbie, Uncle John Piero and Aunt Lucy, Uncle James and Aunt Cori, all of them were our emotional support. They supported and loved Alex, never making him feel different or repulsive.

My mother, Zina, and my father, Joe, and Grandpa Lenny, all have been a huge part of Alex's emotional healing. My mother, was particularly helpful in making arrangements with her priest for Alex to receive prayer sessions. Everyone in the family, including Alex's cousins, Brennen and Reisa, made Alex feel comfortable, no matter how many weird noises he made.

So why move away from such a strong support team at our side? At the time, I really thought that we had no choice. We had to escape the parents and students that were making Alex feel like an outcast, Even his teachers treated him differently once they were told that he had Tourette Syndrome. Children parents and teachers watched his every move, and the more they would stare, the more Alex would tic.

Our arrival home each school day was even worse. He was exhausted from fighting off the tics throughout the day, causing dark circles under his beautiful blue eyes. I begged him to stop trying to hold them back, to ask the teacher permission to go to the restroom and let them out. But Alex explained that he couldn't just take a walk and let the tics begin, because once he let them start, he couldn't stop. Once he stopped trying to hold them in, he would start moving his head back and forth, jerking and barking for hours.

When Alex was at home, he didn't feel that he had to try and hold back the tics. He would bark, and move his torso while his head would jerk and hit his shoulders. Soon after the tics would begin, his head would begin hurting. I think at that time, when he was only nine years old, he didn't realize the severity of it. He believed it would just go away someday, and never come back.

At times he looked happy, even though he was ticing, but most of the time he looked sad. He continued to be close with his brother, Dillion, because being with Dillon was his safety net. No matter how bad the tics became, Dillion didn't care. They were, and still are, the best of friends. Dillion, at such a young age, learned how to deal with Alex and be his best friend. He would hold Alex in his arms and tell him how much he loved him.

My own depression seemed to escalate with Alex's tics. Every night I would pray and ask God so many questions, over and over. I lost my desire to do anything. Even evenings out to dinner came to a halt. My world was Alex: helping him, protecting him and looking for answers. This was my life.

The idea of moving, making a new start, was the only thing that kept me going. I spent a lot of time researching areas and schools; finally, I found a small town in Connecticut that I felt would be good for all of us. The thought of being out of the stress and strain of living in New York begin to fill my days with sunshine. Now Alex would be safe and accepted in a new place. Looking back on my mental state at the time, moving was the only alternative. It was something for me to hold onto, something for me to believe would help Alex.

My excitement peaked after talking with the people at the school, my son would be attending. They assured me that they knew all about Tourette Syndrome, not to worry, he would fit in just fine. This was a school that was equipped with psychology, support groups, and teachers trained to teach kids with T.S. We were thrilled.

The Rose of Denial

In June of 2000, Alex had a new beginning; we had a beautiful new home on a hill, surrounded by roses and trees. It was an exciting time for us. A time that I had created to prove that the grass is greener on the other side. It is interesting how humans have the ability to physically run from their sorrow, only to eventually come face to face with the facts that they were trying to escape.

Our relatives came up from New York to help us get settled. Even though we were all excited and happy about the move, it had created a lot of tension for Alex. His tics began escalating. It was a lot for a little boy in his condition to mentally digest; a new school, neighborhood and home, all in one week.

After three weeks of unpacking and organizing we were finally ready to begin our new life. The first challenge came when Alex and his brother, Dillon, discovered that there was no one to play with in our neighborhood. After introducing ourselves to the neighbors we realized that we had moved into a neighborhood full of retired couples with older children in college. I quickly contacted the principal and asked if she could arrange for Alex to meet some nice boys during the summer. She approved of the idea and soon called me back with the phone number of a boy she thought would be able to connect with Alex.

The meeting was arranged for the mother and son to come to our home. I'll never forget the day. It was a Friday, and we were so excited that Alex would finally have a friend. Of course, the excitement escalated his tics, jerking his head onto his shoulder and barking every five minutes. I gave him his medicine, but it didn't seem to work. I kept reassuring him that everything would be fine, but everything being fine was not an experience that Alex could understand. He had every right to be nervous. His hopes had been trampled beyond repair so many times in the past. I knew the pattern of disappointment had become embedded in his mind, but I had to keep hoping for Alex.

Betty and her son, Carl, arrived that Friday. For once in a very long time, Alex was able to experience the joy of having a friend. The boys played for four hours while Betty and I visited. Betty's husband was a doctor, so it was comforting to be able to talk to another mother who understood the challenges that Alex faced.

The proverbial ball kept rolling, and before long Alex met two brothers through a second meeting arranged by the principal. Then to my surprise, we suddenly had two more invitations from our new friend, Betty, to go swimming at the local country club. I politely bowed out of the first invitation, thinking that it might be another type of stuffy social scene that had been the cause of our frustration in New York. But the second time she called I couldn't say no. I couldn't let the past get in the way of our new beginning.

When we arrived at the country club, the pool was filled with children of all ages. Alex's face turned beet red with embarrassment. I could see his thoughts turning to fear of rejection. We looked around and finally found Crystal and her two boys, sitting at a picnic table. Soon, Alex and her boys were off and running, swimming and playing basketball.

After a few hours, Alex came back to the table and told me he was tired and wanted to go home, so we said our goodbyes and headed for the car. Once we were on our way home, Alex started crying. I couldn't believe it. He had appeared to be having so much fun. He told me that it was the kids that didn't know him that wouldn't talk to him. Even though his new friends introduced him to the other kids…no one talked to Alex. They simply ignored him.

While listening to my son describe his feelings of being abandoned by the other kids as they swam to other side of the pool, became my feelings. I became Alex, feeling his pain to the depth of my being as he said, "No matter how nice I am, Mom, no one will ever like me because of my Tourette stuff. I was in the pool ticing, flapping my head back and forth, and making barking noises, so how could anyone want to be around me?" Deep down inside, I knew he was right. The anger swelled inside of me. I hated them all. I hated society and their kids. Alex was helpless and I was devastated.

Blake and I tried to reassure Alex that the tics would get better, and that we would keep looking until we found the right medicine for him. Alex was 10 years old, at that time, and was taking a drug called, Clonodine, which seemed to help at night, but gave him severe headaches if taken during the day.

The summer quickly passed, and we again reached to the stars, making our wish for a positive school experience for Alex. But that wish soon became a dark star when I found that Alex's beginning into the 5th grade would be attended by a teacher without knowledge or experience with Tourette Syndrome. This was a far_cry from the assurance that the school had given me about the experience of their teachers being able to handle this problem. So, the only thing I could do was to educate her. I gave her photocopies of information on Tourette Syndrome, obsessive compulsive disorder, and Attention Deficit Hyperactive Disorder. She promised to read and study the material.

Life began to settle into a routine for a few months, until the day that Alex asked if I would take him to school, rather than him riding the school bus. I was hoping that he would be able to make friends on the bus, but after questioning him he told me that the kids didn't want him there. I asked him why he thought such a thing. "Because Mom, they put their backpacks on the empty seats, when I get on the bus, so I have to ride in the back of the bus. No one wants me there."

The next day I drove to the bus stop and sat there watching the kids get on and get their seats. Alex was the last one on the bus. He walked up and down the aisle, and finally took a seat in the back of the bus. From that day forth, I drove Alex to school and picked him up. He was so happy and I was happy that I could spare him the embarrassment. But the truth was that Alex was totally segregated. He was an outcast on the bus and in school. He was desperately lonely.

Soon after I began taking him to school he asked if I would come to school and eat lunch with him everyday because no one would sit next to him at the lunch table, and no one would play with him at recess. Before agreeing to go to school to eat lunch with him on a daily basis, I wanted to find out what was happening with him at recess. The next day, I decided to go to school and station myself in an area where Alex would not be able to see me during recess.

I watched the children coming into the school yard, laughing, and playing with each other, but I didn't see Alex. Eventually, he appeared at the door and slowly made his way over to some boys playing ball. He stood there for a few minutes, trying to interact with them, but soon moved on to another group. I watched the same thing happen over and over when Alex would try to interact with the kids, but to no avail. He was right, no one would talk to him.

I battled this injustice over and over in my mind. America, land of the free, where the majority of children seemed empty of compassion for the mentally and physically disabled. Maybe we were just in the wrong place again. Maybe we should move away; look for a more understanding environment for Alex. But, how long could we keep looking, running from what we couldn't change?

Nothing seemed to be going right for Alex or my husband. Blake's search for employment that offered him the amount of money needed to support his family came to a dead end. The following year we sold our new home and moved again, and again I was certain the next place would be the place where we would find a better life for Alex

I was beginning to feel like our life was nothing more than a group of birds migrating from one place to another, feeding our young, and keeping them safe and warm. But, the new city wasn't safe and it certainly wasn't warm.

Alex was to enter the sixth grade in Mt. Carmel, New York, at a very large middle school: My husband and I made our conference rounds with the regular and special education teachers. We finally came to the decision to put Alex in mainstream science, history, cooking and gym, along with resource math and reading.

We felt that this plan would keep him from being shunned and ridiculed. Our plan was only another hope, not reality. But to me, it made perfect sense. The kids would see him in regular classes and would give him a chance to make friends. The plan was a disaster for Alex.

My expectations in thinking sixth grade children could understand a mental disorder that the medical profession couldn't even understand, could only come from the mind of a frantic mother. And 'frantic' was what Alex and I had both become. I couldn't rest, or settle into an acceptance, watching my son breaking apart, inside and out.

The truth is that Alex had violent tics that erupted into strange sounds and movements that very few adults or children had ever seen. But yet, somehow I expected them to understand, to reach out to my son...to know that his tics were not the real Alex. Ironically, the city we had moved from, just ignored Alex, but now we had moved to a place where the children bullied, taunted and teased him, constantly.

As soon as I discovered how the children were treating him, I scheduled meetings with the teachers. Much to my surprise they already knew what was happening and gave me their heartfelt apologies. It seemed that they had tried to stop the mistreatment of Alex by giving the "nice boys" a firm talking to, but after a couple of weeks the bullying began again. There was no end to it.

At that point, metaphysically speaking, I had begun to mentally break away from my body. My heart was broken. There seemed to be no end to my depression, as I tried to find meaning in my life, keep up my appearance, or find solace in my relationship with my husband It all seemed senseless. I was down, spent, nothing seemed to matter. And then it hit.

I began feeling heaviness in my chest. I thought it was just a simple case of bronchitis. But it lingered month after month until one night I woke up feeling like something was ripping in the bottom of my breast, towards the left side; allowing water to go inside of it. I could actually hear it. I couldn't breath very well or lie down on my back. I woke up my husband Blake and had him drive me to the nearest hospital.

I was diagnosed with an autoimmune disease that can attack any part of the organs. The doctors had no knowledge of what had triggered the disease, but thought that it could be environmental. After days of testing they finally operated to remove water from my lungs. I was actually drowning in my own fluid.

The whole experience was torture for my husband and the boys, especially for Alex. His tics were horrible. He cried every night while sleeping in my bed, next to my husband. My other son, Dillon, was only nine years old at the time. He would lay next to Alex and desperately try to comfort him while I was gone.

During my time in the hospital the bullying seem to worsen for Alex. And when things went bad for Alex, Dillon took it upon himself to be there for his brother. I'll never forget my husband telling me about the day Dillon got off the bus and walked to our house. Normally I would have been there waiting at the bus stop, but this time I was in the hospital. When Dillon found neither of his parents waiting for him, he thought I had taken a turn for the worse. When he rushed into the house he was happy to be greeted with a big hug from his Dad, assuring him that Mom was doing better.

But, Dillon knew something was wrong when he didn't see Alex. Blake sat down with Dillon and told him that Alex was in his room, embarrassed and saddened by trouble he had faced at school that day. Blake told Dillon that three boys had thrown food in Alex's face, during lunch that day. He had it in his hair and on his clothes. Before Blake could say another word, Dillon interrupted Blake, telling him to stop. "I can't listen to this anymore, Dad. Just let me go upstairs and be with Alex."

Dillon ran upstairs to his brother's room, and opened the door without knocking. Blake followed behind, stationing himself outside Alex's bedroom door. Dillon walked over to Alex. He was laying face down, crying, his body constantly moving, arms and leg kicking. Dillon leaned over and whispered into his brother's ear.

"I love you Alex, no matter what."

Alex quickly turned over and grabbed Dillon and they hugged and hugged, holding each other for several minutes. Dillon assured Alex that the boys were idiots and just didn't know the real Alex. My husband stood outside the door crying, listening to Dillon telling Alex how much he loved him, and loved hanging out with him no matter how bad his tics were. "We're best friend forever, Alex, no matter what."

Dillon didn't understand Tourette Syndrome, but he did understand his brother. His idol. His best friend. After an hour of talking, the mood changed for Alex and they were soon playing video games, laughing loud, and just being brothers.

Dillon recently felt the need to write a poem for Alex, a poem that comes from a young man who is joined at the heart with his brother.

MY BROTHER ALEX

If you're not from my family, you don't know my brother.
His habits and rituals really are like no other.
Like all other brothers, he does give me stress,
But the difference is, he has Tourettes.

You can't know my brother, his actions surreal.
You can't know his problems, they make grown men kneel.
His problems, so many, no time to heal,
His problems so different, you can't possibly feel.

You think you may know him from movies and shows,
But you can't know my brother, because I barely know.
His feelings, his thoughts, his pain like no other,
Only one truly knows him and that is my mother.

She comforts and loves him with infinite might,
Her strength so incredible through his never ending fight.
You can't see his problems, you don't have the sight.
You don't have the power to make his wrongs right.

Alex's problems so horrible, his pain, oh so deep,
I think he has run out of tears in which to weep.
You can't know my brother, his talent so stunning,
He keeps his wit, as strengths keep coming.

What he lacks in knowledge, he replaces with art,
It is clear, his illustrations do come from the heart.
You don't know my brother, but here's a good start.
Your don't know my brother, but this poem is a part,
of my feelings for him, that come from the heart.

New Horizons

I returned home to my family after nine days. My husband, Blake, was concerned about my chances of a relapse, which prompted us to move out of the bitter New York winters to the sunny skies of Florida. So after the school year was over, we made our way to the land of sun and surf. I now believe that what happened to me had everything to do with my feelings for what Alex was going through, my self pity, and my guilt and shame in believing that my genes had brought so much pain to my son. I had taken that thought to bed with me, every night, for three years, crying myself to sleep. This is what happens when you hold everything inside.

We moved to Palm Beach Florida in June and bought a home seven minutes from the ocean, surrounded by palm trees. Alex loved it. It was a visual paradise for all of us, but I was not fooling myself this time. I had come to realize that there was no magic cure for Alex. But fragile as they might have been, I could not turn loose of my hopes for Alex that someday he would be tic free, and happy to be alive.

Alex tried going to school for a very short time. But, he just couldn't do it. His tics were terrible, so we started searching on the internet for a good private school. We thought at least half of them would be suitable for Alex, since they advertised that their schools were equipped to handle learning differences such as Autism and ADHD, although none of the schools mentioned Tourette Syndrome in their advertising. Tourette disorder is like a hidden disorder. No one wants to talk about it because no one knows what to do with a student who has it.

I always had to educate the teachers about the Tourette Syndrome. Today's teachers are educated in several disorders, like ADHD and autism, but it is rare to find a teacher that is educated about Tourette Syndrome. Alex is now 18 years old and I am still explaining it to teachers. I am looking forward to the day when a teaching degree includes a certification in the education of mental disorders in children.

Alex was rejected by all of the schools on our list, except four. Their comments were usually about the same: "Oh! He has Tourette"? Isn't that the cursing tic? "The truth was that money couldn't buy schooling for a boy with severe tics. But we kept trying. At last we found one that was terrific, in the sense that it had small classes with three highly qualified teachers per class. We loved it, but we couldn't afford $45,000 a year.

It's not supposed to be that way. Every child with disabilities should be able to have the same opportunities to have the best care and education. The search continued with three more interviews in one week. We interviewed with one principal of a school for learning differences, that included ADHD. Everything went well, so they asked us to bring Alex in so they could evaluate him for school.

On the day of the evaluation, after 40 minutes with the Principal, Blake and I knew it was not going to work out. The principal had some nice things to say in the beginning, and we were pleased with him. However, once he told us that Alex was on a trial basis, we were completely speechless. We ask him why our son was on a trial basis and he stated, "Parents pay a large amount of money to educate these kids. I want to make sure that they are not distracted by your son's noise and movements." Blake told the principal that he thought the school was for children with disabilities. "That's correct, but not Tourettes."

Suddenly, his secretary came in holding a file with Alex's name on it. The file revealed that Alex's tics were severe while taking the test, jerking his head and making weird noises. The Principal tried not to show his feelings, but it was obvious that Alex was not welcome. We met Alex in the testing room and told him we were going home.

I told him that the school was overcrowded. Too many kids in one class. "You can't learn that way." He knew something was wrong, and he knew it was his Tourette's. One minute we were loving the school and couldn't wait for him to start, then the next day I'm telling him it's too crowded. My heart was broken. The schools wouldn't help him and the drugs were making him worse.

Soon I found another school with the help of the internet. The photo looked good and I loved their mission statement. It was a school with a mission, educating teens with learning differences, how to learn in a different way by making them feel comfortable in their environment. But the part that really caught my eye was their guarantee that they did not discriminate any type of disability, or race and color.

The school was gorgeous. It had beige stucco siding with a huge water fountain in the middle. Very impressive entrance to the building. Palm trees everywhere! The staff was so pleasant that I suddenly lost all doubts about their honesty. The visit began with a positive note, in that Alex felt comfortable with the principal. After meeting his teachers, it was agreed that he would start class the following Monday.

The principal gave me a list of supplies to buy, which included a school uniform of a white polo shirt with school logo and khaki pants. Alex was so impressed. "This school makes me feel important, Mom. The teachers and principal was nice to me, even though my tics were bad, with the barking sounds. They didn't make me feel different, at all, Mom."

I had also found a new doctor for Alex. After the first visit, it appeared that he had the experience to treat Alex with the right medications. Alex's tics began getting better. A new doctor, a new school, and new hopes. It seemed that we had finally found the niche for Alex.

The first day of school arrived. Alex looked great in his new uniform, so proud, not wanting to let his tics out, holding back, determined to be normal for the first day of school. I tried not to think about what he would be experiencing that day, only to wish him the best, but over the years his fears had become my fears, and being positive had become a lost art for me. Determination, faith, and hopes, were all in place, but not the true peace of mind of that positive "knowing" in your heart that all is well. Alex turned to me as he opened the car door, smiled, his eyes twinkling, "Don't worry Mom, I'll be fine."

That afternoon I arrived at the school about 10 minutes early. I wanted to have time to prepare myself. I was so excited to see him walk out, but was also afraid what I would see in his eyes. It was a constant battle fighting with myself to believe the best. The bell finally rang and I saw teenage kids laughing, talking and playing around with each other as they walked toward their parent's cars. It was a vision that had become my prayer, a day when I would see Alex tic free, hanging out with the kids, happy and laughing. But at that moment, it was all about dealing with the reality of Alex waking me up from that vision, knocking on the car window, "Mom, open the door!" I leaned over, unlocked the door, and looked into the eyes of a smiling face.

Our drive home was quiet. I didn't want to ask him too much, so I just casually asked him how his first day played out. "Good," he said, with a smile. "Mom, It's just my first day, but I did sit with a group of kids that spoke to me at lunch." There was that smile again. I was ecstatic!

Alex made it through one week. We were so proud of him, and especially the school. We took him out to dine at the restaurant of his choice. It was our weekend to celebrate, and celebrate we did. It was a fun weekend, and one we hadn't seen in a long time. When Sunday night arrived, my husband and I went in Alex's room to say goodnight. There was his uniform on the dresser, neatly folded, shoes ready by the door next to his book bag. He was happy again and suddenly I caught a glimpse of something positive.

The next day I drove my happy son to school, never expecting the day to end as it did. Something happened that afternoon. I received a phone call from the principal's office. The secretary told me that the principal wanted to arrange a meeting with my husband, and me. I told her we could be there the following morning. I called my husband and told him, but he didn't think it was going to be anything serious. The next morning we took Alex to school and went straight to the principal's office. Finally we were all seated and ready to discuss what I prayed would not be another problem.

The principal sat across from us, a slight smile but a stern look in her eyes, and then the words came. "First, I want you to know that Alex is a super kid, a very polite young man. But his tics are horrible in class. His screaming and his violent tics are frightening to the students. The movements of his head jerking and arm throwing are disrupting the class. All of them come to this school with attention deficit problems, so when Alex tics, it distracts them. I'm so sorry, we just cannot continue to have Alex attend class here."

The long second that we sat there stunned, speechless, soon exploded into a mixture of sobbing and yelling. I had never seen my husband so angry. It was like a symphony of horror without a conductor. My husband was screaming at her. "You lied to us! Why did you take Alex, in the first place? This is a school for learning differences. You lied to us and made us believe that our son belonged here. How dare you?"

I stopped crying and tried to calm my husband down. I knew Blake was right. Everything he had yelled at her was the truth. But, right or wrong, it was another ending for Alex. We walked out of that office, knowing that our son would again feel alone and humiliated. Once again, we had to explain to our son that his tics were too severe, loud, and too frightening to be included in class participation. When would this injustice end?

At the end of the day, we sat down with Alex and told him what the Principal had decided. He didn't understand, and why should he? The school that had made him feel important, had taken him in with open arms, was now saying that his tics were too loud, too frightening. We tried to let him know that it wasn't his fault, and even though there was nothing that we could do to change the decision, we could, and did, assure him that we would find another school. We were not going to give up. Alex wanted, more than anything, to graduate from high school, and we were determined to make that happen.

Out of a school's fear of a loss of money and prestige, a child was thrown aside by a school that didn't take the time or concern to find a solution to the problem. Alex's reaction to their decision evolved into a night full of violent ticing, body slamming and higher doses of medication, just to get him through the night.

Blake and I lived in a subdivision called Evergreen. The community was very nice. When Alex felt well enough we would go to the fitness club with Dillon, for a little basketball fun. On one of our outings, Alex made friends with a 13 year old boy with Asperger's disorder. The union between the two boys led me to meeting his wonderful mother, Sheryl. After sharing my latest school trauma with Sheryl, she suggested that I interview with the Christian school that her son was attending.

"It doesn't look so hot from the outside, Marina, but the teachers are great, plus they're moving to a new building. Will Blake mind Alex going there since the school is Christian?"

"Are you kidding, Sheryl ! Blake doesn't care where Alex goes to school. Right now, we haven't even been able to find one that will accept him." It was nice to have another woman who understood my problems. I couldn't wait to get home and tell my husband the news. It would be a relief to know that we would not have to go searching for another school again.

The school was small, but they were willing to take Alex, and that was good enough for us. For the first six months Alex's tics were better, but eventually they escalated to the point where we had to raise his dosage. This would cause him to either sleep too much or have terrible side effects. At that time he was taking 100 mg of Zoloft once a day, 2 mg of Clonidine at bedtime, and 10 mg of Abilify once a day.

The medications made him sleep better, but his tics grew worse. They were so bad that he had a lump on the lower side of his head from slamming his head to one side all day. So, the doctor raised his dosages again, causing him to sleep day and night. There were some days that my son couldn't get out of bed.

But somehow, someway, Alex forced himself to finish the school year, through all his self injuries, changing medications, and hating the school he attended. Ironically, one of the reasons he hated the school so much was their policy of making Alex stay in class. No matter how badly he felt like passing out, they wouldn't let him go home. They thought that he might be faking it.

I am always amazed at the warped logic that is frequently displayed by school teachers and administrators. Faking it? He weighed 160 lbs. He was 6 feet tall, very pale and tired looking, as well as being extremely drugged. He had bruises on both sides of his lower neck from slamming his head against his shoulder. What part did they think he was faking?

The end of the year finally arrived. We were smiling from ear to ear, preparing to celebrate Alex passing into the 10th grade. But we were wrong. The school decided to make him do the 9th grade over again. They pointed out that he had missed a lot of class work, and tests, while being out sick. We were shocked. We had always sent a doctor's note when he was absent. They never told us that he would be held accountable for a disorder he couldn't control.

What happened to their responsibility to make certain that he would get his credits to move on to the 10th grade? We were always up front with them, making sure that they knew we would help Alex make up his work at home if he had to be out, even though there were days that he was unable to sit still. He went to school, a mental and physical mess, almost every day because we assured him they would understand and pass him to the next grade. Now our life shifted into another phase. Alex wanted to die. It had all become too much. He just stopped caring.

————————————

Moments of Truth

As it turned out, it was our last summer in Florida. Again the eagle flies, only this time it was going West. A close friend of my husband's, invited Blake to come to Texas to partner with him. Blake couldn't refuse a salary double what he was earning in Florida. At that point there was nothing for any of us to regret leaving, so off we went to Texas. We loved Dallas so much that we bought a house next door to our friends in Plano. Lori, Michael, Regina and Brent, and Jennifer and Kevin, who were doctors, all treated us like family. It seemed that we had finally made a move that had brought us peace of mind and heart.

The summer was over before we knew it and suddenly it was time to enroll our youngest son, Dillon, in middle school, and Alex in high school. Alex had several weeks to get use to the idea of going back to school. He had heard many nice things about the school, but Alex was terrified, paranoid, which I attributed to the high dosages of Abilify and Zoloft, which were also making him gain weight.

He was two weeks away from starting school, so for the rest of the summer we went swimming everyday. Then at night, it was hot tub time for the guys. Blake and Dillon and Alex would sit in the hot tub at night, talk and relax. A great way for the boys to bond with Dad.

Alex started school. A new school, and a new doctor. The doctor decided to keep Alex on the medications he was taking, then he told me the same thing that I had heard and lived through what seemed like a million times: "If Alex's tics get worse after starting school, we'll try a different medication." Never once had a doctor told me that he or she knew what to do, knew exactly what pill to give that had no side effects, or sat down with me and discussed the side effects. Alex had become a testing ground for pharmaceutical companies.

As the school year progressed, we noticed that Alex's tics were evolving into full force mode. Now I know the reason. The Abilify had backfired. After being on it for 3 years, it had run its course, and just like using too many antibiotics builds up an immunity to their effectiveness, so does the excessive use of neuroleptic drugs also lose their effectiveness. At that time, Alex was still on Abilify, Zoloft, and Clonidine.

Clonidine, a drug given to adults for the treatment of high blood pressure, is also found to be useful in the treatment of alcohol, opiate, and nicotine withdrawal syndromes, attention-deficit/hyperactivity disorder (ADHD), and Tourette Syndrome. The fact is, that as of this writing, there is no specific study comparing the use of Clonidine in children with its use in adults.

Clonidine works on specific nerve cells in the brain that are responsible for lowering blood pressure and slowing the heart rate. The side effects are: dizziness associated with sudden changes in body position, dry mouth, constipation, nausea, daytime sleepiness, weakness and lethargy. It was apparent that Alex possessed all of them.

The side effects from Abilify are as follows: fever, stiff muscles, confusion, sweating, fast or uneven heartbeats; uncontrollable jerky muscle movements. Is this another way of saying "tics?" I have asked myself over and over why my son would be prescribed a medicine for his bipolar problem that could cause jerking of his muscles, when he already has tics that caused jerking of his muscles.

Here are the remainder of the thirty two side effects listed for Abilify: sudden numbness, weakness, headache, confusion, problems with vision, speech, or balance, increased thirst or urination, loss of appetite, fruity breath odor, drowsiness, dry skin, nausea, vomiting, convulsions, thoughts of hurting self, feeling faint, jaundice, choking, trouble swallowing, anxiety, insomnia, and weight gain.

As you can see, many of the side effects nullified the drug's initial action to correct the disorder, creating more havoc with his body and mind. Often, it was impossible to tell if it was one of the drugs making him tic more, or the ADHD, OCD, Tourettes, or the bipolar disorder. Since the three drugs had overlapping side effects, it was impossible to determine.

The third drug prescribed was Zoloft. I now call it the "killer drug." According to information posted by the law firm Parker, Waichman, Alonso LLP, in December of 2006, the FDA announced that antidepressants prescribed to young adults are risky. After the FDA completed a bulk evaluation involving 100,000 patients and 11 antidepressants, including, Zoloft, it became clear that there is elevated risk for suicidal thoughts and behavior. In 2001, 1,883 children, ages 10 to 19 years old, committed suicide. The remaining side effects of Zoloft are: dizziness, nausea, agitation, rapid heartbeat, sleepiness, tremors, vomiting, coma, stupor, fainting, convulsions, delirium, hallucinations and mania. Now you can understand the determination and agony my son went through to attend school.

As his tics continued to get worse that year, we were told to continue to give him the Abilify. His doctors kept saying that it wasn't the Abilify making him tic worse. But what about the school and social phobias he had developed? The doctors never mentioned that it could be the side effects.

All that year Alex cried day and night. He missed his cousins, aunts, uncles and grandparents. He could feel himself falling apart, one pill at a time. I could certainly understand his need to be part of the whole family again. Who better to have by your side when you have given up? Alex wanted to go back to New York. His life was nothing but a daily nightmare of side effects, and for what? He was never treated to achieve healthy results. He was treated to dull his mind and body. The medical profession has failed to look at the fact that everything we think, drink, eat, and breath affects specific organs in our body. Neuroscience now has proven that negative thoughts create toxins in our body, and positive, happy thoughts make us healthy and strong. All of the drugs Alex was being prescribed were creating a world of negative thoughts that were, in turn, causing side effects in the body, including serious weight gain.

Mothers and fathers that are in this type of situation want to scream, run away, (and some do), take antidepressants, drink and smoke anything to dull their pain. Many of them become as sick or desensitized as the child. So where do I lay the blame for this legal chemical torture of children with mental disorders? Well let me put it like this…I have a friend that interviewed a Texas senator about laws that should be made or discontinued. He told her that if the people demand a law be made, or demand a law be dropped, it is ultimately up to the people if it gets passed or dropped. It is up to parents to bring change to the way drugs are prescribed to our children.

I believe a law should be passed that requires doctors to try alternative remedies before prescribing adult drugs for children. I believe we can change how doctors treat children with mental disorders, and I believe that school nurses can educate parents with "Special Needs" children on what to eat and drink in order to achieve a healthier mind and body. It is apparent to me that prescribing prescription drugs is the easy way out for most doctors who just do not have an answer or a plan to find the answer. So until we can get a law passed to change this problem, it is up to parents to find alternative counseling and treatments.

Alex's weight gain continued to spiral upwards to 270 pounds. Depressed to the point of talking about suicide, and developing agoraphobia (among many other phobias triggered by the drugs), my son refused to leave his room. I had never seen him just give up completely. We tried everything to cheer him up. Even our friends played a part by inviting him to dinners. Our dear friend Mike, whom Alex thought of as an uncle, tried to coax him out of the house with tickets to basketball games, fishing trips, and swimming, but nothing worked.

Since the men didn't have any luck with Alex, my woman friends began their mission to get Alex out of the house. Regina began with the soft motherly approach, finally turning to more of a sister mode, with no success. Then appeared my good friend Lori, whose professional position gave her access to the Dallas Mavericks events and tickets. She was sure she could get Alex out of the house to go see the games. Well, we all went to the games, and everyone enjoyed them except Alex. Mentally, he was still sitting in his room.

The final step for Lori was to get all of the cheerleaders to sign a calendar, especially for Alex. The result? He smiled, said thank you, but life had waned for him. Breathing, laughing, going and coming-all pointless movements in a pointless world. Again, his pain became mine. He had shutdown and I could feel myself doing the same. The more depressed Alex became, the more I withdrew from life.

I stopped putting on makeup or fixing my hair, even though I lived in a community that sparkled with beautiful women. What others looked like, or did, no longer mattered. I think the unconscious thought of failure of being unable to heal my son, was truly at the root of my depression. I felt defeated, lost in a maze of doctors and drugs that had, for years, brought us nothing but misery. Now, any medical hope we once had for his recovery had faded into a fragile memory.

I was so afraid that Alex would commit suicide. He had talked about it earlier in the year, and often brought up the subject in the middle of his morning panic attacks. Every morning, for seven months that year, Alex's counselor, Mrs. Stone, God Bless her soul, would wait for him at 9:00 a.m. at the main entrance of the school, open the car door and talk him out of the car as he sweated profusely, so afraid that the act of breathing was near impossible. It was a horrible and traumatic thing for anyone to watch.

The doctor had little to say, other than that there wasn't much that could be done that had not already been done, other then to change Alex to a different drug. We wanted to think about making that decision, but our fear that it would just be another drug with another side effect, stopped us in our tracks.

I did feel that I needed to tell the doctor about Alex's threats of suicide, but when he suggested therapy, I informed him that Alex was getting counseling and help at home. Over the years, we had periodically reached out for psychiatric therapy for Alex, which just added to his list of drugs. I had no desire to follow that road again. The doctors should have guided us to obtain family counseling and educated us in the advantages of getting cognitive behavior therapy for Alex. Mental and physical disorders in a family affect the mind and body of everyone. Can they really expect the drugging of one child to fix the whole family?

The school agreed to cut Alex's hours, allowing him to leave at 1:30 p.m. each day, but nothing helped. We knew we had to do something fast. The thought of suicide kept racing through my brain. How long could he live through this physical and mental hell? I finally decided to stop looking for ways to heal him, and search for ways to bring him some sort of long term, or short term peace of mind and heart. It was time to sit down and listen to what my son had to say.

Our discussion led to the same wish that Alex always expressed, "I want to go back to New York." I knew I had to give in to his wish, or lose my son. I could feel it in my heart. He needed to be around his aunts, uncles and cousins, where a circle of love surrounded him, creating a diversion from his anxiety and endless pain.

THE MAGIC CIRCLE OF LOVE

We arrived at my parent's home in Massapegua New York, greeted by family and friends, brimming with tears of joy, and words of comfort. They were all shocked to see how much weight Alex had gained, and the deep sadness in his eyes. But within the hour we saw something in Alex that we thought we would never see again. He was smiling from ear to ear, followed by a flood of laughter, and joking.

He sat next to his Grandpa, Joe, and joked for hours. Just three days before, he had wanted to kill himself. What was different? He was still jerking and barking, but his energy had changed to match the joy and vibrations of love around him. He was around the family unit he had known from birth. He felt safe, at last.

I glanced across the room where my son, Dillon stood silently smiling, watching Alex joking and laughing. I knew by the look on his face that he was happy for his brother. Although I knew Dillon didn't want to move away from his friends, he never complained. He knew he was blessed with a mind and body that was perfect, and so he never questioned any sacrifice that he had to make to give Alex a little peace. You see, watching someone in your family go through years of physical and mental horror does something to your mind and heart. Some people can endure it by constantly searching for any solution that will give that loved one even a small sense of relief, and some people run away.

We had waited until the end of the school year to leave Texas. When arriving in New York we rented a beautiful house on a lake, only 10 minutes from my parents. Alex and Dillon would sit outside, feeding the ducks and swans that wandered into our backyard. The wheel of life seemed to be turning again, full of family, kids and laughter. Maybe Alex was right. It was obvious that this circle of family love had given him great peace and joy, especially his little cousins. Jordan was 4 years old and Maddox was 1year old. Alex was crazy about them. They were so wide eyed and totally accepting of his tics and barking, always bringing up the bible passage in my mind, "be ye like little children." Oh, if only we could all open our hearts and bring ourselves to have that acceptance of others.

Every other weekend, my cousin, Lucy and her husband, GianPiero, and their beautiful daughter, Sabrina, would sleep over at our house. It was great fun. They helped us settle into the house, along with my sister, Debbie, who made my life so much easier. She set the whole house up for me, worked with the movers, and organized the kids' bedrooms. She wanted Alex to feel comfortable as soon as possible. Alex now had the luxury of having his family for breakfast, lunch, dinner, and weekends. He was never alone. His wish had been granted. He had created the perfect diversion from his misery.

Sometimes we would take Alex for a weekend to visit my husband's family, a short twenty minutes away from our house. Aunt Cori, Uncle Jaime and Grandpa Lenny all lived in the same house, near Alex's best friends, Brennen and his sister Reisa. Hanging out with Brennen and Reisa made Alex feel normal. They had known about his Tourette Syndrome since he was first diagnosed, so it was easy for them to overlook his jerking and barking.

I think the highlight of Alex's weekend excursions with the family was time spent with his grandpa Lenny, who was a constant source of laughter for Alex. He's just a funny guy, and to this day, Alex always loved to mimic him.

Summer seemed to fly by. Suddenly I was left with a mere four weeks to get the boys ready for school, Alex in 10th grade and Dillon in high school. Alex's tics were still extreme, and he was still taking the same drugs. I couldn't ignore the fact that there was a distinct possibility that the panic attacks would begin again, the day we drove him to school. I couldn't take that chance, so I decided to take Alex to visit a well known psychiatrist who specialized in Tourette Syndrome issues. I had known about her for years, but the last time I had tried to get an appointment for Alex, she refused our insurance. Visiting her on a cash basis was out of the question for my husband, or ninety percent of most parents.

I decided it was worth another phone call. I told the receptionist that I needed an appointment and immediately told her the name of our insurance. There was a short pause, then a polite, "please hold." My jaw stiffened. I wanted to grind my teeth, claw at the table. Every nerve inside of me was poised, ready to explode. The polite voice returned, casually giving me an appointment date. My God, she had accepted the insurance. At last, I had finally landed the best of the best. I couldn't wait to tell my son.

The appointment was set for two weeks before the beginning of school. I couldn't stop my mind from chattering, over and over, assuring me that this woman psychiatrist was the one. It was time. Alex would finally get the help he needed. He would finally be free of the severe symptoms of this hideous multifaceted disorder.

The day arrived. There we sat across from the famous doctor, my husband, his father, Alex, and myself. She smiled, looking confident, and why not, with 20 years of Tourette Syndrome experience under her belt.

Alex kept touching things in her office. His obsessive compulsion was fired up and quickly becoming out of control. He was trying so hard not to bark. It was like watching one out of control disorder trying to control the other one.

Doctor B. didn't take her eyes off of Alex. She just kept writing and observing, listening to our story and watching Alex. I was so nervous that I exhausted myself, so Blake took over where I left off. We told her the whole story, year after year of trials and errors, sickness and the never ending pain from the side effects of drugs. It seemed odd how we could fit it all into one short 60 minute period.

She continued the session, this time talking only to Alex as he kept walking around the room, ticing, head jerking, barking, and waving his arm above his head. It was like he was conducting his own private symphony. She continued asking trite, mundane questions that even Alex found strange for a high priced psychiatrist. They were all questions he had heard over and over with each new doctor, assessing and prescribing another drug to see if it would fit.

"Have you ever wanted to hurt yourself?"

He answered with a sarcastic tone, then mellowed out. "Yes, how did you know? Yeah, I think about it all the time. In my mind I want to die, but my heart won't let me do it. I guess I love my family too much...can't seem to leave them.. I think it would kill them. I'd rather just take it to the end!"

My father in-law never knew that Alex had such thoughts. The word was out now. Everyone in the family would know. Maybe that was as it should've been all along. I felt my husband's hand on mine, trembling. We couldn't believe our son had accepted a 'cross' that he thought he had to carry for us.

"You have a terrific boy. I think it's time to talk about medicine. Tell me what he's taking now and in the past."

When I gave her the list of medicines that he was currently taking and those he had been on in the past, along with all the side effects that he had to endure, she was stunned, commenting that he seemed to have terrible reactions to medications that are used for severe tics. I sat straight up in the chair.

"What do you mean? Are you saying that you don't know of anything that will help him?"

"Marina, when tics are severe, everyone goes with the traditional neuropleptics, which are, Halperidol, Orap, and Fluphenazine. Obviously, we can't give any of them to Alex."

We were sitting in front of the guru of Tourette Syndrome and she was telling me that she uses the same drugs that all the other doctors used. We were at the end of our rope. At the time, I believed that there was no other place to turn, so tearfully and fearfully, I had to let her try. Her plan began with weaning Alex off of Abilify, and onto Fluphenazine, a drug used to treat psychotic disorders. No, he wasn't psychotic, but she said it is also known to decrease both motor and phonic tics.

Her next step was to switch him from Zoloft to Celexa, which is used for depression. She thought it would be good for his anxiety, and certainly worth trying. Trying? It seemed to always be about "trying" and never about having an answer. This was her specialty, or was it? Obviously, specializing in a subject that has been boxed, labeled "incurable" and stored on a mental shelf, doesn't inspire any effort or possibility of a cure, so the whole treatment becomes nothing more than a symbol of the story of Dr. Frankenstein's trial and error, always hoping his experiments would result in a normal human being. Only, I am the one who was put in the position to be Dr. Frankenstein's assistant, testing, trying, experimenting with my son's life, watching him twist and turn into moments and movements that were ungodly in every way.

We followed her instructions, weaning him off of one drug, adding another, and watching his tics get worse. They were so bad that he would tic all day and all night until he became so exhausted that he would finally pass out. Once again Alex was faced with not being able to go to school. It was impossible for him to concentrate.

Alex was torn apart emotionally. Through all of Alex's horrible years, he held on to his dream of finishing school. He insisted that he had to graduate high school, no matter what. But again, the road was blocked. We had a meeting with the school and agreed to have him home schooled until Christmas, then slowly transition him back into his classes.

School started that September and Alex began his home school tutoring with a fantastic teacher. Ms. K. worked with Alex two or three days a week, depending on how he felt. The complexity of the reactions caused him to be alert one day; moody and depressed the next day. She was astonished at the magnitude of suffering he was enduring. She had seen all types of mental disorders in children, but had never seen a child with self-injury tics.

By that time, we had weaned him off of Abilify, and substituted it with Fluphenazine. In five days of giving him a low dose of 2.5 mg a day, we saw a negative difference in Alex. He developed a new tic of pouting. His lips would pout all day. It looked so weird, something we had never seen Alex do. My past experience told me that the new drug was the cause, but we continued to give him the Fluphenazine for another four days, until he begin making rolling motions with his fingers, nonstop.

I stayed up late that night researching the new drug and found that it could possibly cause a permanent neurological disorder called Tardive Dyskinesia, with a side effect that described exactly the same movements that Alex was doing. I immediately called Dr. B. the next morning, explaining what was going on. She was silent for a moment, and then asked what I knew about Tardive Dyskinesia. I told her I did some research and it seemed that Alex fit the criteria.

She didn't seem to want to discuss it, other than to tell me to immediately stop the drug and bring Alex into the office the following day so she could see for herself. I believed that she knew it was Tardive Dyskinesia." She had to know. My God! She was a psychiatrist, a specialist that is suppose to know how neuroleptic drugs affect people, what to give and what not to give.

We arrived at her office the next morning. Her first question to Alex was, "Alex, since you started taking the new medicine, what did you notice happening to you?"

"Well, my head jerking stopped, but now I do this pouting and rolling my fingers all day."

The session continued with Dr. B. listening and writing as Alex answered her questions. The result was a decision to put Alex back on the Abilify, but to go on with the plan to wean him off of the Zoloft, replacing it with Celexa.

There was no reassurance from her that Alex didn't have Tardive Dyskinesia, but she kept staring at him like she knew he had it. I could tell by the expression on her face. We left her office, preparing our minds for another round of drug experimentation. I wondered when this would all end. What would be the ultimate ending of this horror show?

We started weaning Alex off of 125 mg of Zoloft, which would have normally taken a few weeks, but her instructions were to start giving him the Celexa when we had him weaned Alex down to 75 mg, and continue until he was completely off of it. Three weeks later Alex started acting impulsive, screaming nonstop. He couldn't sit still because his legs would shake constantly smacking into each other. It had to be the Celexa. I wanted to call Dr. B. and yell obscenities at her. Twenty years of experience, specializing in Tourettes, and she couldn't help him. Another dead end.

Here we were, back in New York with our family, seeing who is suppose to be the best doctor in this field, and Alex is no better than he was when first diagnosed. From that moment on I started praying every night, the same prayer I had been saying from the first day Alex started having tics. Often, at night, my mother and I would go into his room and pray over him. He loved the inner calmness it brought him.

We took Alex back to Dr. B. She took one look at him and gave instructions to take him off what she had prescribed and put him back on what he was taking when he first went to visit her. Through all of this hell of side effects, Alex still wanted Ms. K. to tutor him. He still wanted to learn and pass to the next grade. He would tell his father and me that he wanted his tutor to teach him the same lessons that the other kids were learning. I asked him how he could learn anything with his tics being so bad. His answer was that there were kids in the hospitals with all kinds of things wrong with them. Some of them have tutors, so if they can learn, so can I. I'm not sure where he found logic in that thought, but it was enough for us to continue his tutoring.

I asked Ms. K. if she thought that Alex was truly learning. She assured me that he was retaining the information she was giving him. She wasn't worried about the days he was unable to read or write, because if his tics were too bad to read and write she would do it for him, then review the work and ask the questions.

The majority of the time his answers were correct. The only time Alex had a lot of trouble with his school work was when it came time to work on his math. Math stressed him considerably, bringing on a stream of tics, but somehow he would pull through it with a passing grade.

I think the love connection between Alex and his teacher, and their drive to overcome the extreme physical obstacles, made them a rare team. We were all blessed to have her working with Alex.

———————

IN THE SHADOW OF DEATH

We had been back in New York for about four months when I realized how much life takes on a lighter note when the love of family surrounds you. My sister, Roseanne and cousin Lucy would often visit, bringing their children. Somehow, their presence made our life seem easier. It was always an escape for Alex. A moment in time when he was treated like everyone else. Everyone in the family did all they could to make Alex feel better, but his tics just kept getting worse.

Two weeks before Thanksgiving, Alex developed a new tic. He would swallow and then burp out the air, over and over, louder and louder. My sister Debbie and her husband Brian had invited us over for Thanksgiving, so when the day arrived we were excited and happy to get out of the house.

Our families ignored Alex's tics, so we had a beautiful dinner, but that night Alex started acting shy, and going to the bathroom a lot. After while he wasn't talking at all, which, for Alex, is unusual. My sister even played his favorite rap song, then we all got up to dance to our type of music. After about 30 minutes I realized he was not in the room. I looked for him, but didn't find him anywhere within the mass of friends and relatives.

I asked Dillon where his brother has gone and he told me Alex had gone up to the bathroom. Five or ten minutes went by and I decided to go up and check on him. I knocked on the door, but there was no response. I waited quietly for about five minutes, then I heard him throwing up. No amount of knocking on the door would get a response out of him. I was yelling and banging on the door so loud that my sister came running up the stairs. She got a tool to pop the door open. When it opened we couldn't believe what we saw. There was strange looking vomit everywhere.

Alex then told us that he had been vomiting for a week. We cleaned him up and went home, but soon after we put him to bed, it started again. The next day I called my mother to get the phone number for her gastroenterologist. We called the doctor and made an appointment for that Monday.

On Monday morning my mother and sisters came over to help me get Alex ready. They looked at him and started crying. He looked pale and weak. He was sweating and ticing through it all. My sisters helped me get him dressed and pack all his medications. They were upset, but they gave Alex hope. They told him, "Don't worry, Aly boy. You're okay, we promise." He didn't respond. He just looked at me with terror in his eyes. I tried to look back at him with hope in mine.

We all got ready and headed off to the hospital. Alex was in the front seat with my husband; the rest of us were in the back seat, praying. My son started vomiting digestive blood into a plastic bag. My sisters begin crying silently crying, trying not to show their faces to Alex. I prayed hard: "O Heavenly Father, God of Love, You gave us your son, Jesus, to be physician of our souls and healer of our bodies and minds. Lord, I turn to you in this time of illness. Please go to Alex and lay your healing hands on him. Let the warmth, peace, and healing power of your spirit heal Alex today." The hospital was only 30 minutes away, but the drive seemed to last forever. We hit every stoplight.

My brother-in-law, Allen, called me to give Alex some encouragement. He knew Alex couldn't talk, he just wanted him to listen. I put my phone on speaker and told Alex that Allen wanted to talk to him. Allen said, "Alyboy, you are going to be all right, you hear me? I don't know why this is happening to you. But I love you and I will pray for you. Hang in there, man! You're my hero, Alyboy!" We all cried. We didn't expect Allen to call us at that moment. Alex was so emotional that it made him tic more.

We finally arrived at the hospital. My husband drove around the circular driveway and let us out. Once we got out we noticed that Alex was bleeding from him mouth. The blood was all over his shirt. It must have started as soon as we pulled up to the hospital. Blake parked the car and met up with us. As soon as we walked in, we registered Alex. The staff immediately took Alex into a room and started examining him. Blake and I were terrified, looking at our son with nurses all over him. The rest of the family was waiting and praying in the family waiting room. Dr. G. finally came in around 11:15 a.m. They drew blood, urine and a little bit of stool. Alex was horrified. He just wanted to go home. The tiny room we were in was so cold, so sterile. A pink curtain was drawn around us. Blake and I stood next to our son. The nurse gave Alex a bed pan in case he had to vomit.

After two hours, the doctor walked in with test results in his hands. I felt like I was going to faint. It was cold inside the room, and rainy and freezing outside. The weather was horrible that day. It felt like we were in a nightmare. The doctor told us that the good news was that Alex was not hemorrhaging anywhere in his body. "Oh, thank God," I said to Blake as I grabbed his hand.

"No, but he does have digestive blood coming from his stomach."

"Why his stomach?" said Blake.

"Well it's not coming from his nose or lungs, but there is blood in his stool. I want Alex to have an upper endoscopy and an upper GI."

He wanted to do all this in two days. He told us that Alex could go home, but we needed to get him to the hospital the next day and schedule the upper endoscopy. A week later they would do the upper GI series.

We had the first appointment in the morning. Alex couldn't wait; he was up the whole night. He stayed up with me in the family room. He was not allowed to eat or drink after midnight; he hadn't been able to eat the whole day, anyway. My father-in-law was there. He was so nervous that he watched TV with us the whole night. We all told Alex that it was going to be a very short procedure and then the doctor would give him something to stop the vomiting. Nothing made Alex happy. I didn't blame him. The thought of the procedure made him even more sick. He threw up throughout the night. I felt like crying and telling him I wished I was going through this instead of him.

Finally around 9:00 p.m. we settled down to watch a funny movie. We laughed a little, and after the movie he fell asleep on the couch. I didn't have the heart to move him, so I left him there and slept right next to him on my chair and ottoman. I watched him sleep all night. I knew that the next day he would be terrified, but he looked so at peace in that moment. It was wonderful seeing him like that, but it didn't last long.

We had to wake him up at 6:30 am. Our appointment was for 9:00 a.m. but they wanted us there early. We arrived at 8:15 am. When we got to the hospital they took Alex in while Blake filled out some insurance forms, then met us in the operating room. We were all telling Alex over and over again that it wouldn't hurt and he wouldn't remember anything. He just sat there, looking at me, with two big tears rolling down his face.

The doctor explained that the I.V. would just hurt for a second, then he would get sleepy. He said, "OK," with a trembling voice. She let us stay with him until he fell asleep. He was shaking so much that he needed two nurses to hold him down. At that point they told us to kiss him goodbye because he was going to go out any minute. His eyes closed and out he went. We walked back to the waiting room. Blake and I barely spoke. I prayed the whole hour and a half. The procedure was only 90 minutes, but he would need another hour to recover.

After the 90 minutes had passed, the head nurse came out and told us that everything had gone well. She brought us into the recovery room while Alex was still asleep. A few minutes later the doctor arrived. She said that Alex's stomach looked great, and his large and small intestines were clear and clean. The only thing she found was that the bottom of his esophagus was raw; she said that some of his tics had caused that problem, and that was where the blood was coming from. She said she had also done a biopsy on his stomach and would let us know the results in a few days. She gave us Nexium to give him two times per day. We were relieved that one test was over; now all that was left was the upper GI series.

Alex soon began waking up. He was groggy. I touched his face. I was always amazed that he could keep going through one drug calamity after another.

"Mom?"

"I'm here son, it's Mom."

"I love you, Mom."

"I know, but I love you more, sweetheart. Daddy is here with me."

Blake kissed his forehead and told him everything was OK. Alex asked why he had been throwing up blood. We explained to him what the doctor had explained to us. The doctor came to him as soon as Alex was up and talking. She told him what was wrong and he understood. Once Alex had gathered his strength, Blake helped him get dressed. I went to get the post-op papers for him. The doctor gave me Nexium and her card so we could call her for refills. She reminded us not to expect any miracles in the first week.

Alex slept in the car all the way home, while I caressed his arm that the IV had been in. He was just relieved it was all over. Our families were waiting for us at home. They couldn't wait to see him. They all had balloons and "get well" cards for Alex. His bed was freshly made, waiting for him. My sisters had washed and sterilized everything in his room. Everyone, particularly Dillon, was thrilled to see him. Dillon just cried and hugged his brother. Blake and my father, Joe, walked him upstairs and put him in bed. Dillon sat on the floor right next to him. Our families didn't stay long; they understood we all needed some rest. My father-in-law finally was able to get some rest, too. He was so worried he didn't sleep or eat until we got home with Alex. I couldn't sleep even though I was exhausted, so I went out and bought the foods the doctor had told me to give him. Alex did a little better that night. The next day was even better. He was still vomiting, but it was not as bad as before; I think he was more comfortable knowing he was going to be better.

We still had the upper GI series to worry about, however. The doctor wanted to make sure that the small intestine was not blocked. Alex had to drink eight bottles of this horrible white chalky stuff, so the doctor could ensure that it passed through his small intestine. He was not happy. He cried, "First they stick a tube down my throat into my stomach. Now they want me to drink this shit and take pictures of me drinking it." That's exactly what they did. They made Blake and me wait outside in the waiting room. The doctor told us that if the chalky stuff stopped halfway through, then there was a blockage of some kind. The doctor said it could take up to six hours for the chalky liquid to pass all the way through. Three and a half hours later the nurse came out to get us.

The doctor told us first that Alex was fine. The milky stuff had passed slowly all the way to the bottom. They took 30 pictures from the beginning to the end. The doctor then went on to tell us that Alex was one of his favorite patients. He was cooperative and kind, and did everything the radiologist told him to do. He drank the shake without a fight, and smiled the whole time. Everybody loved Alex. Teachers, nurses and doctors said the same: he has been robbed of his childhood, but he still manages to smile and be funny. Alex got cleaned up. When he came back out to us he said, "Let's get the hell out of here. I'm fine, Mom."

When I got home, Grandpa Lenny told me that Dr. G. had called. My father-in-law was relieved that Alex was fine. I was nervous, so I had Blake call the doctor back. The news was great: no stomach cancer! Alex was perfectly fine. The vomiting was less severe because of the Nexium, and the blood had completely stopped. Thank God!

Still, the vomiting was a problem, and we had to figure out why it persisted. After two weeks with the same symptoms, I called the doctor. She said, "Give it time. The Nexium needs at least a month or two to work." We waited, continuing the Abilify, Zoloft and Clonodine; now we had to add Nexium.

Alex was still being home schooled. There was no way he could attend school. Alex hated that he could not go to school and lead a normal life. One night in the midst of all this, as we put him to bed, Alex said, "Mom, don't feel bad for me please. I still have good thoughts left in my brain. It may not look that way sometimes because I am going through hell, but the good thoughts are in the back of my head. Whenever life gets me down, I go back to those little thoughts and know that I'm going to be fine and free. I know I'm going to beat this, I just know! Please forgive me if I ever snap or yell at you and Daddy and Dillon. That's not the real me."

———————————

Thinking Into The Light

Alex once told me, "The worst thing is when people pity me. It makes me feel terrible. I don't want that and I don't need that. I just want the same things everyone else does. It's just harder for me than for other kids. I just want these horrible tics to go away so I can finish school. I want to graduate, Mom. And I will! My problem is I have no friends. I never grew up with friends. When I did go to school, kids thought I was crazy and weird. They either make fun of me or ignore me. I wish they could get past that. But they can't!"

Alex was still regurgitating his food. I continued giving him Carafate once a day, but we had gone from three times a day to once in a period of three months. I was still in contact with his pediatric gastroenterologist, but he wasn't getting what I was saying to him about Alex. I would call and update him on Alex's condition every three or four weeks. He always told me to give Alex Carafate three times a day, and that he would get better soon.

One day in the middle of winter, I was in the home office staring out the window. Alex was downstairs working with Mrs. Kamen. I turned to my computer and started doing some of my own research on Alex's regurgitating. I just knew it wasn't normal. I was happy all the tests showed that he didn't have cancer, but something wasn't right. I couldn't get help from his doctor. I found some web pages on food allergies and the side effects they can have on people. I found out that a gluten free, wheat free, and yeast free diet could help, so I decided to try it.

I went to heath food stores and started buying Alex wheat free, gluten free, yeast free food. I started giving it to him a little at a time to see if he could digest it. The first day I made him a plate of pasta with a little extra virgin olive oil and sea salt, he did not throw it up. I thought it was just a coincidence, but that same day at dinnertime, I made him pasta again. This time I added some organic peas. I thought "Oh, no way. He'll throw up. It's too heavy." He said, "Mom, you're giving me peas? You know I can't eat vegetables." I told him to try a little of it and see if he could tolerate it. Much to our surprise, he ate the whole dish. Hours went by, and he kept his food down. I was thrilled with the change. I thought it was too good to be true.

In the weeks to come I gave him organic carrots, organic spinach, organic string beans with organic chicken and turkey. I started cooking wheat, gluten, yeast free pasta. He wasn't throwing up anymore. No more smell of vomit from his breath. No more regurgitating his food. It all stopped. Alex had been vomiting digestive blood, regurgitating while he was on medication. Suddenly Alex was not regurgitating at all. He was eating three meals a day. I couldn't believe that changing his diet would have such an impact on him. I started buying everything from snacks to meat as long as it was gluten, wheat, and yeast free. It worked!

We also started noticing that Alex had fewer tics. Dillon told me that ever since we had changed his diet, Alex was ticing less when they were together alone. When Dillon told me that I wanted to cry. Was changing his diet a tic reducer? How could that be? After three months of that diet he was no longer vomiting. I started documenting everything he ate, and how he acted right after. My husband and I discussed with Alex the possibility of slowly wening him off his medications. Alex was thrilled. He had been waiting for this day to come.

I called Dr. B. and told her exactly what had been going on. She didn't show any emotion at all. She just said, "I don't think it's the food, but I'm happy that Alex is doing better." I told her that ever since we had changed his food he had been better. His regurgitation had stopped and tics decreased. She said she thought that maybe finally Alex was growing out of his tics. I did not agree. I saw immediate change in Alex as soon as we changed his food. She told us if we decided to take him off his medications we had to go very slowly, one medication at a time. We were thrilled. We started with the strongest one of all, the Abilify. We started giving him 5 mg a day instead of 10. The 150 mg of Zoloft and .2 mg of Clonodine stayed the same. In the first few days we did not notice anything. That was good. We continued with 5 mg for the rest of the week. The second week we maintained the same dosage.

In that second week, we noticed that Alex started acting strangely. For one thing, he was having a lot of trouble sleeping. Although he was not vomiting anymore, or barking or throwing his arms in the air, he had developed new tics. He would constantly move his head side to side and almost hit his shoulders. The motion gave him terrible headaches, and it was difficult for him to concentrate on school work. He also started twisting his jaw. When we got him down to 2.5 mg of Abilify, the new tics worsened. We knew that after five years on Abilify, the withdrawal would be difficult. Once we had weaned him completely off the Abilify, the jaw twisting became almost unbearable.

One night he was in a lot of pain, and finally showed Blake and me the inside of his mouth. I looked and saw what appeared to be two huge black holes. Alex had damaged the lower back inside of his jaw by scraping and biting it with his back teeth. Apparently Alex had learned to tolerate pain so well that he didn't even know when something serious was wrong with him. Blake went out that night to buy an ointment for canker sores. We thought that would help. I put gloves on and gently put the liquid on Alex's sores. I then gave him two Motrins for pain. By that point he had begun to cry. I told him that he would feel better in a few hours. Alex had always had canker sores in his mouth, but nothing that ever looked like this. He went to bed right after that. I was hoping he would sleep through the pain and wake up feeling better.

Later that night he came up to our room again, crying. He just kept saying, "They hurt and I can't stop. I can't stop!" My husband and I asked him what he couldn't stop. He said, "The more it hurts, the more I have to bite down on it and grind my teeth." I got up and walked him to his bathroom while Blake went for the Motrin. I put on another pair of gloves and gently spread more ointment on his sores. It hurt him terribly even to open his mouth halfway for me, but I managed to apply the medicine with a cotton swap. Finally, we took him back to bed. I could see Alex was in a lot of pain, so I stayed with him for the rest of the night. I rubbed his head and prayed over him. Eventually we both fell asleep in his bed.

Dillon woke me up at 7:30, getting ready for school. Blake was so exhausted he hadn't even noticed that I wasn't in bed. I got out of Alex's bed and walked over to Blake and Dillon. Blake asked me how Alex was. I told him he had finally fallen asleep around 3:30. I told Blake I was starting to worry about the sores in his mouth. Blake reassured me, "He always gets them. They will go away. They just take some time."

I didn't bother waking Alex for Mrs. Kamen. He needed his rest. I took a quick shower and drove Dillon to school. Dillon asked me, "Mom, is Alex going to be OK?"

"Why are you asking me that?" I asked.

"Because he's always sick," he said. "There is something always wrong with him. I feel so bad for him, and for you. I've never seen you like this, Mom." I couldn't believe he was speaking to me like this. "Mom, you look terrible. You don't take care of yourself. You've lost so much weight. You don't do your hair anymore. All you do is cry."

He was right! I hugged him hard and told that I loved him. "Things will get better somehow, someway," I promised him. He looked into my eyes and nodded, and stepped out of the car. I watched Dillon walk away and open the school doors. I started to cry as I realized that my beautiful healthy boy was suffering now too. His grades were dropping. He did not get much sleep; none of us did. He was so worried about Alex and me that he took it to school with him. I sat in the car and prayed aloud: "Heavenly Father, a Father who cares for me, who provides for me, who protects me. Oh my God, I believe in you. I hope in you, I adore you, and I trust you. Have mercy on all the mothers of this world and grant them a true spirit of motherhood, that they will love and cherish the children you have generously given them. Please help me through this, God!"

I cried the entire drive home. I knew that once I got inside, I had to deal with the pain Alex was going through. When I opened the door I was met with silence. I called Alex's name but got no response. I called again: nothing. I ran up to his room, opened the door and saw Alex sleeping face down. I walked over to kiss him. When I bent down to kiss him on his forehead, he was burning up. I quickly went to my medicine chest and pulled out the thermometer to check for fever. I gently woke him up and told him that I was going to take his temperature. His eyes were still closed. He was mumbling something about pain. He had a fever of 103 degrees! I ran to his bathroom for Motrin. When he got up to take the medicine, I saw that the right side of his face was swollen. I asked him to open his mouth. He did, and I saw something repulsive. He had a gigantic black hole in the side of his bottom cheek. We had not fully realized how big the sore was the night before. It was the size of a half dollar coin. Alex was in so much pain that he couldn't speak. He started to cry. I felt helpless. I told him to stay in bed and let the Motrin kick in. He did while I called Blake and told him to come home right away.

Alex could not sleep. He got out of bed and started pacing back and forth with his hand on his cheek. I tried to keep him calm, but it didn't work. He started screaming. I couldn't understand: I had given him Motrin 1 ½ hours ago. How could the pain not have stopped? I couldn't wait until Blake got home. I didn't call my family; I didn't want to worry them. My heart was pounding so hard I could literally hear it. The worst part was he continued to tic through the pain. I t was bizarre. The more his mouth hurt, the more he had to bite the sores. It was terrible! I tried putting ice on his cheek, but he wouldn't let me. He said I couldn't touch it. I walked away for a few minutes to calm myself. I heard the front door open, and Blake came running upstairs to Alex's room. Blake called out for me, "Marina, where is he?"

"He's in his room, Blake."

"No, he's not."

"Yes he is, Blake."

We both were surprised to find him in our bathroom. He was looking into our mirror, crying. Blake grabbed him and said, "Alex, let me look at your mouth." When he did, he was as shocked as I was. "How did it get so bad?"

Alex cried, "I don't know, Dad, I don't know!"

Alex started to pace again. He looked like he wanted to crawl out of his skin. I asked him to stop pacing so I could take a good look in his mouth again and saw that his cheek had doubled in size over the past four hours. His mouth looked as if a boxer had punched him. We didn't waste another minute. We took Alex to the emergency room.

On the way, I called my sisters Debbie and Roseanne to tell them what was happening. They were quick to offer help and said that they would take care of Dillon. Then I called my cousin Lucy to ask her to pick Dillon up from school. I told her what was going on, and she started to cry. "How much more pain can this boy go through?" Then she said, "Don't worry about Dillon. We'll all take care of him." Thank God for my family. I couldn't have made it through without them.

Alex was scared and in throbbing pain. We told him not to worry, but we were all scared. The drive to the hospital was horrible. We had just done this three months before; I could not believe it was happening again. Alex was sitting in the front, holding his cheek and crying in pain. He couldn't sit still enough to put a on a seatbelt. Blake was speeding to get him into the ER. By the time we finally got there, I was shaking. Fortunately the ER staff took Alex in right away. They took his temperature and blood pressure; both were very high. A nurse started drawing blood. Alex had a hard time keeping still, but he managed to cooperate for a moment. She then wanted to take an EKG, but she couldn't; he was ticcing uncontrollably. His body looked like he was being tortured. His head would slam onto his shoulder and then he would scream in pain. Then he started kicking his legs. He was kicking everything in the room nonstop. After 45 minutes, the doctor finally approved morphine for Alex. As parents, we were miserable to watch our son endure the worst pain he had ever experienced. I kept looking at my husband for support. We didn't know how his sores had gotten so bad.

Blake kept looking out from our room to see if the doctor was anywhere in sight. Finally, he walked in and told us what was going on. He was young, but seemed to be very knowledgeable. First he took Alex's temperature and blood pressure again. Both were still high. Alex looked terrible. He was sweating profusely, his eyes were closed and he was screaming in pain. The doctor was holding Alex's chart. Blake got up out of his seat and spoke to him while I sat next to Alex, drying the sweat from his face. The nurse took my blood pressure too; she said I didn't look well. I did feel like I was going to faint. I sat and prayed silently to calm myself. The doctor told us that Alex's red blood cell count was at 18,000.

"What does that mean?" I asked.

"It means he has a horrible infection running through his body. From the looks of it, it's coming from his mouth." He said he'd never seen a sore that was so big and caused so much damage. He told us he wanted to give Alex antibiotics intravenously, and that if the fever did not go down he wanted to admit Alex to the hospital for the night. My heart was in my throat. Blake started crying.

"I want you guys to understand that even though I believe the infection is coming from his mouth, I need an oral surgeon to look at it, immediately. So right now let's try to get the fever stopped and give him some additional morphine."

As soon as the doctor stepped out of the room, two nurses walked in. One started the antibiotic and the other changed the sweat-soaked sheets. Alex was incoherent the majority of the time. Periodically, he would beg us to take him home. Blake assured him that we wouldn't leave him alone, but he had to stay just a little longer. I sat next to our son, drying his forehead and face, while Blake massaged his shoulders, hoping that Alex would fall asleep for a few hours. Then every time the morphine started to wear off he started ticing, crying, and screaming in pain.

After 4 ½ hours in the ER, Alex's fever finally started to respond to the antibiotic. The doctor checked in on Alex every 45 minutes. The doctor told us he had found a great oral surgeon right next to our house. Our appointment was made for 8:00 the next morning. The doctor told us that if he had not been able to find an oral surgeon so quickly, he would have admitted Alex to the hospital. They checked his fever one more time: 98.6 degrees. Normal. The ER doctor took down our phone number and all of the medications Alex was on.

A few minutes later Blake listened as the ER doctor put a call into Dr. B. to discuss Alex's medications. The doctor's response to her concern about the antibiotics was that he needed to get rid of the infection first before worrying about the tics. She agreed. When he came back into the room, Alex was finally asleep. He was still sweating profusely, but his fever was down. Blake let me know that Dr. B. thought that weaning Alex off the Abilify had triggered the biting tic inside of his jaw and cheek. I maintained that the Abilify itself had caused the problems. She told the ER doctor that she wanted to see Alex as soon as he was better.

At last, Alex was allowed to leave. Blake helped me get him out of the sweaty gown. We washed his face, neck and hands, and got him out of bed. He was so happy to leave. The doctor gave me a list of things to do for him when we got home. He said to give Alex two Percacets for pain and lots of fluid. The antibiotics would begin the next morning.

As we were driving home in the middle of the night, I suddenly felt my fear being replaced by determination. We had made a promise to our son, a long time ago, that we would find a way to heal him. I didn't know how it would happen, but I knew I had to keep searching

When we arrived home, his face was so swollen that he could only sleep on his left side. Drugged and exhausted, he slipped in under the covers and drifted off. It would be a short night's sleep for him, and a sleepless night for Blake and me. He would not stop sweating. I knew that was normal because of the infection, but I had never seen anyone sweat so much. I had to change his sheets after three hours. At 7:00 we started getting ready for the oral surgeon. Alex looked terrible. Blake helped him get dressed. He started crying with slurred speech, "Please, I don't want to see any more doctors!" Blake told him he had no choice.

The doctor had him lie down on the chair. Alex opened his mouth and shut his eyes as the brilliant light above revealed the inside of his mouth. "I can't believe it," she said. "I have never ever seen ulcers this bad." I didn't know what ulcers were, and asked her to clarify. She explained that they are like canker sores, but with a break in the mucous membrane. Sometimes they are filled with puss, and they fester and corrupt. She said that she didn't have to drain the inside of the ulcers; the swelling would go down with the Percacets and antibiotics. It would take some time, up to three weeks, for the swelling to go down. She was very confident that she could help Alex. The antibiotics were to continue, even though it was going to be rough on his body. The infection had to be stopped before she could help him. Alex was now on capsules of Clindamycin, 300 mg, three times a day. I had a vivid idea where this was going to lead, but tried not to think about it.

Alex was now on heavy duty antibiotics, Percacets for pain, Zoloft for anxiety, and Clonidine for tics. We had eliminated the Abilify. We had all been so happy to take Alex off his medications, and now we could not continue the process. The following days were grueling.

Alex couldn't continue his tutoring sessions because he was in so much pain. The antibiotics brought out the worst of the tics. He was jerking his head violently again, bruising his shoulders. His fingers were swollen from cracking his knuckles constantly. The antibiotic helped the infection but he hated the way it made him feel. Percacets and the sheer exhaustion from ticing all day were all that allowed him to sleep through the pain. Every night for the next week, I would go to his room and wake him up twice a night and change his sheets and his pajamas. He hated it, and I hated to have to interrupt his rest. However, the antibiotic made him sweat so much that it was unthinkable to leave him covered in it all night. Our lives were hellish that week.

My mom, Zina, my dad, Joe and Blake's father, Grandpa Lenny, took the situation with Alex really badly this time. Alex's tics waxed and waned. They had always been bad, and he had no life for eight years—but this past year had been his worst. I think that they had seen enough of their grandson in so much pain. My mother later told me she would cry and pray all night for God to heal her grandson. Every day seemed the same.

Fortunately, my wonderful family was there with me from the moment they found out about the ulcers in his mouth. My mother cooked for all of us. My sister Debbie did the laundry for us. Roseanne and her little boys Jordan and Maddox brought smiles and hope to our lives. Lucy would bring her darling daughter Sabrina to cheer Alex up. Sabrina and Jordan, both 4 years old, and Maddox, 14 months, couldn't have been more delightful. Alex just loved watching them play. It took his mind off his issues. The kids were so gentle with Alex. It's like they knew he was sick. Those kids brought happiness and purity to our home that we will never forget. My terrific brothers-in-law would come over every night to watch funny movies. Alex loved hanging out with them, even when he was in so much pain. My cousin John Luca, who had such a busy life, made time and would drive almost two hours just to visit with Alex. John Luca is very spiritual, and would speak to Alex about God. They would pray together. Alex has never forgotten the love and care that everyone in my family took turns in giving.

When Alex was finished with his antibiotics and the swelling had gone down, my cousin Lucy and my sisters Debbie and Roseanne gave Alex a facial. Lucy gave him the best head, back and shoulder massage he'd ever had. Alex loved that. He always begged Lucy for massages. He said it put him in another world. He also loved Aunt Debbie's foot massage with her special creams. He was in heaven that day. They adored him and gave him that treat because they just wanted to see him smiling and relaxed.

My nephew Brennen slept over as soon as Alex got better. They had a blast. Brennen knows Alex well enough to know when to goof around and when just to relax and watch movies with Alex. Brennen and Alex are the same age. That year they were sixteen. They started kindergarten together. They had been on the same youth baseball team together when Alex had to quit after two months because of the tics. Brennen didn't care. He was like another brother to Alex. And my niece, Reisa – oh, how Alex loved hanging around her! She's two years older than Alex, and she is beautiful. Alex always says he hopes to meet a girl that looks just like his cousin. I tell him that one day he will. She loves rap music, she can dance, and she is very sensitive. Alex was still ticcing badly but trying to make the best of it when his cousins were around.

I took Alex to his oral surgeon for a follow-up visit two weeks after the antibiotics were finished. She said that his ulcers looked much better; he was doing great. Alex was as relieved as we were that the ulcers were healing. She wanted to see Alex again in three weeks to make sure the infection was completely gone.

We were back after one week. I couldn't believe it. Alex's tic of biting his sores had returned. It had been gone for about a month. The antibiotic brought out his worst tics. The oral surgeon couldn't believe Alex was biting his sores again. We explained to her that he couldn't take antibiotics - when he did, things like this would happen. This time she gave Alex an expectorant to swish in his mouth three times a day instead. She told us it would taste bad but that he needed to do it so the sores wouldn't turn back into major ulcers. Off we went to pick up the expectorant; Alex tried it as soon as we got home. She was right: he hated the taste. But we had to try it.

That week he had school again. Mrs. K. started coming over every day. She was so wonderful. She was patient and loving with Alex. They just picked up where they had left off. Alex had missed almost two months of work that he had to make up. Mrs. Kamen told me that week what a fighter Alex was. She said, "I have been teaching kids all day every day for 15 years, and I have never met a student like Alex. Through pain and loneliness and depression, he always seems to have the most genuine smile. How can anyone smile after going through what he does day in and day_out?" I answered her, "He does it with God's guidance and love. God is always around my son."

Another week went by, and Alex's mouth tic was still there. We couldn't believe it. Through it all, Alex still wanted to be weaned off the rest of his medicines. We believed it was the right choice, but didn't want to do it while he was still grinding and biting the inside of his mouth. However, he didn't want to hear anything but "yes" to no more medicines. Finally, we all agreed: No more medicines. He was thrilled.

His stomach got better after we rid him of Abilify. His diet helped with most of the other tics. At this point we believed that after weaning him off of meds, his tics would be a lot better. So I called his psychiatrist to let her know what was going on. I recounted to her the past five weeks we had experienced with Alex. She said the oral surgeon had called her and explained what was going on. Alex's psychiatrist felt awful for him. First the regurgitating tic and then the mouth-biting tic. Then I told her I wanted to wean Alex off of Zoloft and then Clonodine. Those were the only two left. She said, "I think you're crazy! You want to take away the medications that work for him, so he can stop ticing?"

"No," I said, "I believe the medication backfired and he tics more now from his medications." I told her we had changed Alex's diet and had seen some improvement. "Well," she said, "do what you think is best for Alex. But I don't agree with you." She told us to start weaning him off the Zoloft by 25 mg every week. When we finished that, we were to start with the Clonodine. She said to wean him to 1 mg for two weeks, then .5 mg Clonodine for one week, then none. She wished us luck, and told us we knew where to find her. No more psychiatrist! We were on our own.

Alex still ticed badly with his biting. But we still agreed: no meds. By this point we were almost off the Zoloft and Alex was still ticing. I knew being off of medicines would be a roller coaster. The days to come were horrible. Alex was still on the same diet as before: no wheat, no yeast, no gluten. But that's all I did. I was not giving him any supplements or other natural foods he needed because I had just started learning on my own what to do. I knew I had to take him to a homeopathic doctor but I wanted to wait until the tics were almost gone.

While these things were happening to Alex, Blake was working part-time for a local bank as a mortgage broker, but times were hard; homes were expensive and were not selling. With the collapse of the housing market, his income became an issue. Blake put his resume on the Internet, but nothing happened. He tried getting jobs through old friends in New York, New Jersey and Connecticut, but no one had any openings.

We didn't want to leave our families again. But as soon as we had made the decision to return to New York, for Alex's sake, things had started going downhill for all of us. We were struggling financially and trying to cope with Alex's horribly brutal tics. Other than enjoying our families, we hated New York. Blake's employment problems, mixed with Alex's self mutilating tics were becoming more than we could all endure. My son Dillon also became depressed causing a grade drop from A's to C's.

This was not what I had expected to happen when we moved back to New York. My wonderful family was so happy we arrived. They had been so excited we were coming back, and we felt the same way. It was obvious that our destiny was not meant to be in New York. Blake decided to call his old friend Michael, whom he had worked for the year before in Texas. Michael quickly extended an invitation to return.

That meant leaving the family again. It was a hard decision. We discussed it for weeks. As we tried to make an intelligent decision Alex still had the same mouth tics. He was still getting ulcers. We were constantly returning to his oral surgeon. Eventually she expected us every few weeks. Dr. R. finally decided on a solution to the problem after conferring with another doctor in her practice. They wanted to remove Alex's back top and back bottom teeth. We were shocked. She showed us Alex's mouth x-rays and pointed out the problem.

Dr. R. and the other surgeon explained that if they removed those teeth, Alex would not have ulcers anymore. Even if his ticing continued, he would not be able to hurt himself. No back teeth, no cutting into his cheek or jaw. That sounded great to us. Now we had to tell Alex, who was waiting in the chair in the examining room. I knew that it was going to be difficult to explain to Alex that the doctors wanted to remove teeth, but we had to do it. Blake and I walked into the room where Alex was stretched out on the examining chair waiting for us. Alex looked at our faces and knew something was wrong. He looked up at Blake and said, "What's up, Dad? What's wrong now?" Blake put his hands on Alex's shoulders and looked him the eyes and said, "Alex, Dr. Rosenberg, and Mom and I, all agree that if Dr. R. removes the last two teeth on the top and bottom you will not suffer from infections or ulcers anymore. We think it's a great idea. It won't hurt anymore. It can't! You won't have any teeth cutting in to your jaw or cheek."

Alex was completely shocked. He was speechless. I don't think he really understood the reason until weeks after it was done. At first he was very quiet. After about ten minutes of thinking he said, "Okay. Let's do it." Blake said he would go tell Dr. R. I stayed behind with Alex. He held my hand tightly. He wouldn't look at me, but he started crying quietly. Big tears rolled down his face. He looked so helpless and depressed, but he knew this was something he had to do.

Dr. R. walked in, ready to do the extractions. She asked that Blake and I leave and wait in the waiting room until she was done. We kissed him and told him that we loved him and were proud to have him as our son. As soon as we stepped out of the room, the nurse closed the door and they got started. Alex didn't want local anesthesia, he just wanted the Novacaine shots. He told Dr. R. he was sick of anesthesia.

While I was in the waiting room, I couldn't help thinking to myself, Has God forgotten my son? Or perhaps I was being punished for something I had done in the past. Why was my boy suffering so much? At 16 his tics should had been getting better, not worse. But then I realized at that moment: This was something Alex was born with. Only God knows the plan. Even though Alex's young life had been stolen from him, my son was still a loving, caring, and funny boy. He took his Tourette's with dignity and acceptance. Through all of his torturous tics he always seemed to dream of the brighter picture.

The procedure went well and Alex was soon able to get into the car. We got home that cold and windy Friday afternoon and put Alex into bed. I propped up his pillows like the doctor had told me to do for the next few hours. I then removed his bloody gauze, gave him his painkiller with some water, and gave him new gauze.

Alex rested in bed while Dillon read to him about his favorite hip-hop artist, 50 Cent. I had bought Alex a book about him for Christmas, but Alex was always so sick that he hadn't had a chance to read it. Dillon pulled up a chair, leaned over to Alex, and started reading to his brother. As I walked away to make Alex some soup, I turned around and looked at my boys again. I was fortunate to get that glimpse of the love they have for each other. I thanked the Lord for the two best gifts a parent could have.

Alex's mouth finally healed after four months of ER trips, oral surgeon visits, removed teeth, and lots and lots of painkillers. There we were in the beautiful month of April, and we had decided to move again. This time it was because of my husband's employment problems. We all knew the best choice was to move back to Dallas, where Blake had a friend who wanted to help us. That part was great for us, but I couldn't help feeling horrible for leaving our families again. Alex and Dillon had become so close to their little cousins, Jordan, Maddox and Sabrina. They had been there to cheer Alex up when he was scared and depressed. He loved watching funny movies with Jordan and Maddox, and falling asleep with Sabrina under her fuzzy pink blanket.

We had to break the news to our families. My family had tried everything in their power to help Blake find work in New York. Sadly, even with their love, support and help, He couldn't find anything that would support us. Dillon and I knew the severity of Blake's situation, but we kept it a secret from Alex. I didn't want to cause any more stress for Alex. We told Alex that Daddy was having trouble finding work in New York and that Uncle Michael wanted to help us, but we had to move back to Dallas. Much to our surprise, Alex was okay with it. I think Alex had high expectations when we arrived in New York. I know he thought he was going to be healed once he was with his family, but that didn't happen.

The boys and I spent the rest of the spring and early summer with our families, while Blake flew to Dallas to begin working. Ironically, Alex's tics started getting better, and both boys were excited to get a fresh start. They knew their father would be working, and we could live a better life.

Blake finally came back from Dallas to help with last minute packing and work with the movers. He had been away from us for two months. We missed him so much. We were happy to see him again. Blake said it felt weird, but good, going back to Dallas. He said all of our friends were excited that we were coming back. It would be a very relaxing atmosphere, which is great for Alex. The boys were nervous about starting school, but we told them they had the whole summer to get adjusted and make friends. They were also happy that they would be starting a new high school together for the first time. Alex would be a junior, and Dillon a freshman.

Moving day finally arrived. My sister Debbie had us over for a wonderful last dinner with family. We ate, cried, laughed and cried some more. My mom and dad wished their best to us as a family, giving their prayer and hopes that Alex would soon out-grow Tourette's. They all took turns holding Alex in their arms, taking turns saying goodbye. It was especially hard for Alex to say goodbye. His tics were terrible that night, and he couldn't stop crying. But again, he knew it was the best choice.

The next morning we drove to Blake's sister's house to say goodbye. She made a delicious lunch for us. Brennen, Reisa, Cal, Uncle Jaime, Aunt Cori and Grandpa Lenny were all there waiting for us. As soon as we arrived, there were lots of hugs and kisses at the door. Uncle Jaime and Alex went for a walk with Iggy the dog. Alex loved talking and joking around with Uncle Jaime. Jaime always made him feel very comfortable. He had a way of making Alex calm down and stop ticcing. Cori was upset that we were going back to Dallas, but she was happy for us. She had really tried helping her brother find work, but it just didn't work out.

It broke my heart watching Alex, Dillon, Brennen, Reisa and Cal laughing and fooling around in Cori's family room. They all got along so well. They only knew Alex as their cousin, not Alex with Tourettes Syndrome. Alex could tic and scream and they didn't even care. They truly love Alex.

My father-in-law was sad that we were leaving but knew it was the best thing for us. That day we sat in Cori's kitchen and talked about Alex's funny pranks on Grandpa Lenny. My father-in-law would sleep over at my house all the time, and Alex would always walk into the guest room and joke around with him. Even when Alex wasn't feeling well or had terrible tic moments, he found the time to pull pranks on Grandpa. Alex once shaved Grandpa Lenny's head while he was sleeping. Lenny came down to breakfast with us and half the hair on his head was missing. I know that sounds terrible, but it made Alex laugh all day. We all laughed, even my father-in-law. He said, "How did Alex do it? I didn't even know he was in my room." Another time Alex asked Grandpa if he could fix his hair before we all went out to dinner. Grandpa said yes, of course. Alex used half a bottle of gel. He slicked Grandpa's hair all the way back. We laughed so hard. It took three washings to get it off. Lenny looked like a greasy mobster. Alex just loved pranking, especially Grandpa Lenny and my parents. I think those were times Alex forgot he had Tourette's. It was wonderful to see him have a good time acting like a clown. We have seen so much sadness with him that we accepted his acting like a clown and pranking his grandparents all in good fun.

We had a great day at Cori and Jaime's house, but finally we had to leave. The movers were coming the next morning at 8. My sister-in-law took lots of pictures with the cousins all acting goofy, and some serious ones. They all posed for the camera hugging, with great big smiles. We said our goodbyes. Again we all cried! Alex said to all of them, "Please don't cry anymore. We will be just fine in Dallas." Alex wanted his cousins to visit us over the next school break. They said of course they would. We hugged, kissed, cried and left another family. No one spoke in the car. Dillon was very quiet. Alex was ticcing. He was jerking his head and barking. It was all too emotional for him. When we got to the house it looked so sad and empty. We slept in sleeping bags in one room. I gave Alex 50 mg of Zoloft and 1 mg of Clonodine. We were almost done with his medicines. We couldn't wait. Alex's jaw tic was almost gone. That night we all fell asleep quickly; we were all emotionally drained.

The alarm clock woke us up at 7:00. We took our last showers in the house. We got dressed and ready to close this chapter of our life and start a new one. The movers were at the house at 8:00 on the dot. My sisters came and picked up Alex and Dillon for lunch while the movers were there. They got to spend a little more time with their cousins. I didn't want Alex around anyway; it was just too stressful. He still wanted to be with my family, and seeing the moving trucks hurt him.

The movers had everything out of the house by 6:00. By then it was just a big beautiful empty house full of horrible memories. I closed Alex's door one last time. I couldn't believe how happy we had been to move back to New York, only to leave with such bad memories. I just wish it could have worked. When my sister dropped the boys off everyone was in tears. They walked into the empty, dark house. We were packed up and ready to leave. Roseanne and Debbie and Lucy grabbed Alex and Dillon, hugged them hard and whispered, "Let's not say goodbye, let's just say I'll see you later!"

Blake was ready to lock up the front door. Debbie, Roseanne and Lucy walked to their car, looking over their shoulders until we pulled away in our taxi. Their faces were sad and their eyes were filled with tears. They blew their last kiss to us and drove away. We all got into the taxi that was taking us to the airport, and looked at the house one last time. Then, surprisingly, Alex said, "Let's go now please!"

Alex leaned his head on my shoulder all the way to the airport. Dillon just looked out the window in a cold stare. Blake said, "Guys, I know you don't want to hear this right now, but God has a plan for us and I think he's leading us to them. The Lord has plans to prosper us and not to harm us. The Lord has plans to give us a future full of hope." The plane ride was quiet. Alex hates to fly, but I gave him a sleeping pill as soon as we got to the airport, and he slept all the way to Dallas. We arrived around 1:30 in the morning. When we got there, he was neither happy nor sad. Dillon was even a little happy. Blake and I were optimistic and ready for our next challenge. Blake knew Dallas so well that he knew exactly where to go even in the dark. We had a rental car for one week until our cars arrived from New York.

We all started waking up when Blake was driving us to our new house. It felt strange to be back in Dallas. I have to admit, the Dallas skyline put a smile on my face. By this time we were all getting excited as we neared our new house in Frisco, Texas. The suspense was killing us. We had never seen the house or neighborhood before. Alex started ticcing out of excitement. When we finally got there it was so late and dark that we couldn't really see anything. We pulled into the garage and couldn't wait to go inside. We jumped out and left our bags inside the car. We wanted to see the house. Dillon opened the door to our new beginning. The house was beautiful! It was smaller than the one we had had in Plano, but it was still beautiful. The boys ran up to pick their rooms. Alex got the biggest room overlooking a field of greens. The house was quaint. The boys slept on the floor in the master bedroom with us.

We fell asleep quickly that night, and were awakened by the doorbell ringing nonstop. We must have overslept from exhaustion. The movers had arrived at 7:00; they said they waited almost an hour until we finally heard the bell ring. Blake jumped up and said, "Wake up, guys! The movers are here!" We were all so happy. It took the movers all day to unload the truck and set up the house. They left all the boxes in the garage so we could unpack at our leisure. Alex grabbed his boxes and brought them happily into his room. Dillon did the same. It looked like the boys were happy.

Over the following week we unpacked and organized. We finished the kids' rooms first. I wanted Alex and Dillon to be comfortable in their new house. They seemed to be adjusting just fine. The crazy thing is that Alex's tics were few and far between. By that time I was giving him just 25 mg of Zoloft and had stopped the Clonodine. He was not slamming his head anymore. He was still doing the burping and barking tic, but the body movements had stopped. We didn't want to bring that to Alex's attention because sometimes when we remind him of an old tic he'll do the same tic again. So we watched our son not have body spasms or head jerking anymore. It was obvious that something was working.

The boys made friends with our next door neighbor's daughter, Emman. She is beautiful, intelligent, and very nice to Alex and Dillon. Within a few days, the boys had met Emman's friends, Maddy and Ashley. They come over from time to time and hang out with the boys. Alex loves that. They're great girls! Through the girls' friendship, Alex and Dillon started meeting their friends. Now the boys have Ryan, Emman, Ashley, Maddy, and Daniel. They all go to Frisco High School. It was great for Alex to make friends and relieve some of the pressure he was feeling. They never asked Alex what he has. It's like they already knew. They didn't even ask Dillon. These kids had respect and love. What a great way to start a new high school with good friends.

Alex had a fantastic month before school started. He was ticcing a lot less and meeting new kids that liked him for who he was. He was feeling great! His tics were great. We had completely changed his diet and he seemed happier. He still had some tics here and there but they were nothing in comparison with what they had been four or five months before.

Still, with school starting soon, I began to worry that Alex's tics would return full force. We told Alex about the same thing we always did before going to school, or when meeting new people. We told him we were very proud that he was finally ready to go to school. He was going to walk into a high school and sit in class, do his class work, socialize and make friends.

Before Alex started school, my husband and I had an ARD meeting with Frisco High School. We actually had one over the summer and then two weeks after school started. We explained to them what Alex had and gave them Alex's evaluations from past doctors. We gave them all the information they needed. The ARD meeting was a great way for all of us to discuss what our plans and goals for Alex were. Alex was there at the second meeting. I thought it was great that Alex wanted to be there. Mrs. Vicky_Perkowski, the vice principal, Alex's head teacher, Amy Snowden, Alex's school therapist and the school counselor, Mrs. Shelley Schwartz were all there along with Blake, Alex, and me. We all sat around a boardroom table. I was so nervous. I'm always nervous before the ARD meetings. That's probably because I'd always been Alex's advocate, always fighting for my son's rights. I've had a lot of practice.

However, this time it was different. I didn't have to advocate for Alex. He did it himself. I couldn't have been prouder to see him sitting there like a man in front of very important people and saying what he wanted to say. The staff just loved him. I was so surprised that Alex only had very light tics. I caught myself, at times, holding my breath in awe. Mrs. Perkowski asked him questions that he answered very intelligently. He even helped them choose his own classes. He was calm and very polite in the boardroom with the school staff. He was so comfortable in the meeting that he asked everyone for a favor. The Vice Principal and teachers were eager to hear what he had to say.

"I want everyone here today to tell the other teachers and kids that I have Tourette Syndrome, so I know how to prepare myself for how to answer any questions the kids have. I don't want pity. I just want the same opportunities the other kids have. I have no problem talking about my disability. It doesn't mean that I'm dumb or a freak. It's important that teachers and kids know this. Sometimes you might hear some barking or see some movements from me, but those are just tics, something that I have to live with every day of my life. But Tourettes is not who I am inside. I am separate. I am me!"

We went home that day, and enjoyed a long awaited, peaceful evening. We were so proud of our son. Alex and Dillon got ready for school that night. They picked out their clothes, and found shoes that matched their outfits. I've never seen Alex so happy to get ready for school. It was a blessing from God.

The next blessing came in September Seaon Ducote introduced us to Dr. Constantine Kotsanis. She had studied metaphysical healing and alternative remedies and herbs for years and felt sure that there was a way to stop Alex's tics. I had weaned him off of all medications, and put him on an organic diet, gluten, wheat and yeast free foods, but I knew there was more work to be done to control the whole spectrum of disorders.

After the initial biomedical testing for toxins and allergies, Dr. Kotsanis began treating Alex with nutrition, homeopathy, neural medicines, homeopathic supplements and a special diet. It has been one year since Dr. Kotsanis began treating Alex. He is happy and strong and feels like a new person. Everyone is amazed. It's a miracle!

Alex has a better outlook on life now. He likes going to school and socializing with friends. He suffered with severe tics and depression for ten years. Now there is no more head jerking, no torso movement, no more biting his mouth, and rarely will we notice even the slightest tic. His brother, Dillon, can't believe the change in his brother. Dillon just said the other day, "I can't believe Alex is going to school every day, without tics.

Now Alex can tell you how grateful he is. ***This is Alex's favorite prayer:***
Dear God, Thank you for the gift of keeping me going through the worst part of my life. Thank you for all the many blessings you have given me and my family. Thank you for always protecting me from all sorts of evil thoughts. I thank you, God, for all the healing you have given me and my family. Thank you, God, for the joys and

times I had with my family in New York. Most of all, thank you for the gift of faith that you have given me: the faith to live on.

I'm so glad that Blake made the choice to move to Frisco, Texas. Frisco High School has been one of our angels, providing a challenging and comprehensive curriculum, along with a loving and nurturing environment. They teach their students respect. Their students were very understanding. Alex now has a close friend, Ryan, that he met at Frisco High School. He is understanding and a great friend to Alex. No one has ever made fun of Alex, or even stared at him, at Frisco High.

Mrs. Vicki Perkowski is the vice principal of the school. She was compassionate, understanding and always ready to solve a problem. She is like that with all her students, and their parents. Alex calls her Aunt Vicki. I can't think of a better chief of staff to care for our children.

Amy Snowden is Alex's Special Ed teacher, and like a second mom to Alex during school hours. She takes our children under her wing. No matter what our kids do she is understanding, loving and nurturing. I have called and emailed her countless times on a weekly basis. She always responds quickly and fills me in on Alex's day. Alex has been doing well academically because he loves the school and his teachers, Mrs. Snowden, Mr. Lee, Mrs. Young and Mrs. Jenny Mikeska. They have all been a huge part of Alex's life. It's amazing the joy and inspiration that a good school can instill in a child.

Alex's dream is drawing near. He will be graduating from Frisco High in May of 2010. We are so proud of him. He feels that he has won the victory, and now he can close that chapter of his life. How I wish it was that easy for me to do the same, but as a mother, it is hard for me to forget that my son was robbed of great times at parties, school events, close friends, because of the lack of knowledge the doctors exhibited in treating my son for eight years. It is hard to believe that they chose dangerous drugs for my son, rather than to suggest alternative tests and treatments.

We are all thankful to Dr. Constantine Kotsanis, William Shaw, Director of Great Plains Laboratory, Rhonda Majalca of Integrated Health Research, for treating and helping my son, free of charge. I also want to thank Dr. Mehl-Madrona for extending an invitation to Alex to take part in his healing intensives.

We finally have our son back and it feels great! It would be hard for anyone to understand how far he has come. **Alex always says to me now, "Mom, to those who have experienced it, no explanation is necessary. To those who haven't, no explanation will do."**

Marina is now educating herself in the art of herbal and supplement maintenance.

Family Acknowledgments

To Alex's aunts Debbie, Roseanne, Lucy and Cori – thank you so much for all your help, and for loving Alex so much. Thank you for all your kind words when they were needed the most. For all the late night sleep overs just to make Alex feel happy and loved. He adores you all.

To Alex's uncles, Allen, Brian, GianPiero, Jaime – thank you for spending time with Alex at his lowest point in life. Thank you for making him feel normal, special and wanted. We will never forget that. Cousin Johnluca, thank you for making Alex laugh when it was so hard for him to even pick up his head. Thank you for your kind words and prayers. Alex will never forget you.

Cousins Reisa, Brennen, Cal, Jordan, Sabrina and baby Maddox – thank you for always making Alex feel like one of you guys. Thank you for making him feel like nothing was ever wrong, and for always making him laugh. You're the best cousins in the world to Alex.

Uncle Kamal (screen name Anthony Azizi), you were there when Alex was a little boy. You had such patience, knowledge, and love for our Alex. You moved away from us to become the actor you are today in L.A., but your phone calls to Alex have been inspirational to him. Thank you for praying with and for Alex. He is 18 today, and you will always be in his prayers. He'll never forget you.

How do we thank Alex's grandparents? To my mother Zina, and my father Joe, we love you so much. You have been there for us every step of the way, from the day Alex was diagnosed until today. Your prayers, your tears and your unconditional love for Alex will always be remembered. Alex has a lot of all of you in him. He carries you in his heart always. We thank you.

Aunt Sina, Aunt Rosa, Aunt Nina, Uncle Joe, Uncle Peter – thank you for putting up with Alex's crazy moments. I know he drove you crazy sometimes but he does love you all. Thank you for all your prayers and tears. They will never be forgotten.

To my son, Alex's brother Dillon, you are a wonderful son and an angel of a brother. Thank you for loving your brother unconditionally…always by his side. You are truly Alex's best friend. You have handled Alex's problems better than anyone. You are our Golden Child and a platinum brother.

To our angels that left us so early and now are in heaven: My father-in-law, Lenny, Grandma Ruth, Godfather Frankie and Uncle Saul. We know you will always shine your love down on Alex, blessing him today and every day. Your beautiful spirits are always around us. God bless you all.

TO ALEX WITH LOVE

Dear Alex,

Although you are my nephew, you've always felt like a little brother to me. We fought like we were siblings. I'd sometimes forget that you had Tourette Syndrome. I didn't know much about it at first. You always tried to hold in your tics, as hard as it was, and say you were doing okay with your beautiful smile.

I know you struggled throughout your childhood and always felt like you were different. I never realized how difficult your life was until you moved back to New York in 2007. I saw you at your worst, having been on so many medications almost half your life that didn't work. I couldn't believe all the pain and suffering you were going through. Your tics were constant, as were the regurgitations, the vomiting, the bruises on your body and the anger that you had inside of you because of this ugly disorder. My heart broke to pieces to see you that way. Still, the real Alex managed to come out and make me laugh with your funny jokes and impersonations.

Your face lit up every time I came over with the boys. I think you forgot all your pain and suffering in those moments. The boys love you to death and I know you feel the same about them. It's amazing that because of you, my Jordan, at the age of five, is able to accept and understand children with disabilities. I have learned a great deal from you through the amazing strength and courage you had throughout all this and how much encouragement you gave me when you saw the tears in my eyes.

I want you to know how much I love you. I am so proud of the handsome and intelligent young man that you have become and of how much better you are doing. You are an inspiration to me because you are fighting to beat this disorder every day and moving on to be the lovable person that you are.

With love,
Aunt Roseanne (Rosie)

Dear Alex,

I remember like it was yesterday when you were just a cute little innocent boy who didn't have a care in the world. You became the little brother that I never had. I enjoyed every minute we spent playing video games and going cruising with the music loud.

As time went on and you were getting older, your tics became more visible to everyone around you. The strange thing is, in my eyes you were still my little Alex. I saw past your tics or just didn't want to see them. As time went on, your tics got so much worse. I had no choice but to accept that you had Tourette Syndrome and understand the pain you were going through. It broke my heart every time I looked at you.

If I had one wish, I would wish for you to have had the wonderful life that you deserved. When kids are supposed to be having the time of their lives, hanging with friends, there you were, sitting home, trying medication after medication because nothing made you feel normal.

One thing I want you to know is that you were never alone; you always had me by your side. It's funny how you always looked up to me and wanted to be like me, as if I was some hero. You are the real hero. All the pain and suffering you have been through, the side effects of the different medications, the way you used every ounce of energy in your body to try to hold back your tics at least for a little while so people wouldn't look at you funny – it all proves it. You still managed to put a smile on your face, and on mine.

I hope that one day my two boys have the strength and courage that you possess. I am so proud of the strong man you have become and have shown that you are a true survivor even though to me you are still that cute little innocent boy.

I love you.
Uncle Allen

———————————

To Alex,

Your struggle as a boy, and now as a man, has left my heart broken so many times. I just couldn't understand, "Why does this have to happen to you?" I, myself, suffering for so many years from anxiety and depression, have always looked to you as my inspiration. There were days that, in my presence, your tics would act up more than usual. You would see the pain in my eyes and say, "I love you, Aunt Deb." Well, Alex, I love you, because you are my hero. Your warm heart, your intelligence, your sense of humor and your beautiful face – those are just a few of your best qualities. I know you will fight this fight for however long it takes. Watching you get stronger as the years go by has mended my broken heart.

Your Aunt Debbie

About Alex

Ever since Alex was born, he was the highlight of the whole family. I remember going to the hospital from a disco I was at in my miniskirt and high boots. I was so sleepy but did not want to miss his arrival. I lay down on the couch at the hospital and waited for him to be born. Everyone from both sides of the family was there. When I took my first look at him, I knew I was in love. He was so beautiful, and still is, with those big blue eyes of his and that smile like John Travolta's. Alex is a very sensitive loving kid and very generous; he would give you his shirt off his back and not ask for anything in return. He is family oriented. Maybe we can say that because he has grown up with not many friends. His families are his friends. He was always around us and still, to this day, is close to us. He would come out to dinner with us when he was seven or eight and we would laugh that he wouldn't order a kid's meal but usually a steak. He feels at ease with us and wouldn't have it any other way because kids make him feel uncomfortable about his syndrome and we, on the other hand, let him be himself, tics and all.

I first noticed that there was something more to Alex when he was at my house and was playing outside in my backyard. There was a party being thrown by my downstairs tenants. A lady was saying that Alex was rude and very disrespectful. I was really angry at the woman for talking about my little cousin that way, but I knew that he could not control himself. He was still not ticcing then, but he was all over the place. I remember specifically every time he went to bed he needed to tell his mother "I love you" a few times, and that he needed her to answer back with, "I love you too, Alex." He would reply, "One more time, Mom." When I later noticed Alex and his movements it broke my heart. I did not understand why he was making the noises he was making, and why was he twitching so much? Marina and Blake sat us down one day and explained that he had Tourette Syndrome. We didn't know what that meant. Tourette's in our family? How? All that really mattered was that he was healthy; that's what I kept telling my cousins. In my heart of hearts I was crying on the inside for them. Seeing him get worse and worse, especially this past summer when he was gagging and spitting up blood, was the zinger. We all just broke down and let ourselves go. It was the worst it had ever been, including the times when he was in so much pain from moving his arm or shoulder, or from his neck and jaw movements.

My fondest memories of Alex are when we would sit on the couch to watch TV or a movie. He loves it when I caress his arm or scratch his back. He says it makes him feel better and relaxes him. I do it for hours; I don't want him to suffer more than he *has* to, so I oblige. On certain occasions he can't fall asleep and I go up to his room while he lies down. I scratch his head or his back until he gets sleepy. We discuss his feelings and his thoughts for the day. It's a way for us to bond, and I treasure those moments always. Just like that his tics stop. I marvel at the thought that the only time he is tic-free is when he's fully asleep. A tear drops down my face just thinking that he's a kid that just wants to fit in, in a world that won't let him.

Love Aunt L

Alex
strong and gentle
impulsive and calm
outrageous and private
tough and sensitive
hopeful and dispirited
misunderstood

There is not one memory that I can recall that defines our relationship, but rather all the small insignificant times that make up the big you.

Up until you were about 9 years old I cannot think of you without Brennen by your side. Walking to school together (with Jesse and Norma, remember them?) riding bicycles (Brennen trying to keep up), second grade when you both were in the same class (trouble makers), Queens College camp (what a disaster), little league baseball (remember when you swung the bat so hard that you almost took John Romano's head off?), hanging out with Uncle Jamie, listening to rock-n-roll in his sports car while Brennen was hanging out with Dad talking sports, class pictures, always the tallest and Brennen right beside you (who could forget those cheesy smiles) and then Tourette's. (Brennen never noticed and if he did he never said anything.) You moved far away and broke our hearts, and Howard Beach was never the same to us anymore.

The years following get fuzzy. You weren't around the corner anymore and the times we spent together were few and far between. I remember when you came upstate for the weekend (winter fun), and when we visited you in Florida (summer fun), When you flew from Texas to be at Brennen's Bar Mitzvahs (to be with all those people, old and new must have been difficult for you), I knew the Tourette's were getting almost impossible for you yet you always put on a smile for us. And at the same time you were never inhibited with us.

I miss the old times which are my fondest memories. It's hard to believe you will be 18 years old this March. A young man with a heart of gold and more courage than anyone else I know. I believe that your soul is of the strongest and that is why God has chosen you for this mission. One day you will realize that you were given a gift. I am most proud to call you my nephew. We all have so much to learn from you so I thank you for coming into our lives. Alex, you will always hold a special place in my heart. Always stand tall and lead the way.

All my love,
Aunt Cori

TO ALEX WITH LOVE FROM FRISCO HIGH SCHOOL

I first met Marina Sharfman, along with her sons, Alex and Dillon, in the summer prior to the 2008-2009 school year. I was new to Frisco High School, and to the district, and was trying to appear as if I had my act together enough to start meeting parents. I simply had to rely on my 27 years experience in education (10 of those years as an administrator), and the fact that my background was in theater, so I could always "act like I knew what I was doing!"

Into my little office walked a beautiful, blond lady followed by two very handsome young men. All three had a most wonderful New York accent. Marina introduced me to Dillon, who was to be a freshman in our school. Amazing young man, loves basketball, quiet at times, but I could tell was dedicated to the family and the well being of his older brother. Next, I met Alex. He was a tall, handsome young man, who was a little tentative at the prospect of meeting me. I could tell both young men were a little nervous. Little did they know that I was nervous also.

I have learned over the years that it is most times better to listen than it is to talk, so I listened. Marina told me of several students who had baited Alex into thinking they were his friends, all along, setting him up for embarrassment and heartache. She told me how they tricked Alex into meeting them places, only to stand him up. She continued with the reliving of phone calls received that involved profanity and harassment. As she continued this tale, I looked closely at her face, seeing a mother's love and concern for her child. Looking across at Alex's face, I saw his eyes turn downward, his body get smaller, and his face look so very sad. I saw Dillon's face look at both his mother and his brother with the face of a young man who was at a loss to help protect his brother from such heartache. She communicated to me the reports to the police and the concern that the students involved were going to attend this high school.

I was at a loss as to what to tell her. I did not know anyone and had not met any of the students yet. I could not give her insight as to the school or the students within it. All I could do is feel for her with a mother's heart and communicate to her my dedication to the protection and education of Alex.

I drew from my past years of working with thousands of students. I told her the truth...that bullies usually don't last long and that I have been constantly amazed by the tolerance and acceptance of most teenagers. I shared with Marina, Dillon and Alex the many stories of how I had seen an entire school accept a student who initially thought of never being accepted. I assured her that I would do my personal best at letting Alex know that I was there for him. I promised to make it a part of my daily routine to see Alex and welcome him every day. I assured her the best teachers, the safest school, and the most love Frisco High School had to offer.

I have, and have always had, the idealistic trait of looking at the inside of a person instead of the outside. This meeting was no exception. It was 20 minutes into our meeting that I noticed Alex was ticking. I noticed that as our conversation went on, I was able to make all three Sharfmans laugh and that laughter seemed to lead to a calmness within Alex that made his ticcing start to disappear. As he felt more comfortable, his eyes became bright, his smile became distinct, his amazing personality became apparent. Alex continued by telling me of his love for music and girls. I just had to inform him that it was Texas law that he could not date until he was 45 years old. (Ok, I embellished a little.) Don't worry. He only bought that one for about a nano second! We all laughed some more.

His mother continued, confessing her anxiety with bringing Alex to our school, citing her discontent with his previous schools. She informed me of his medical conditions, his disappointment with his previous educational settings, and her hopes that Frisco High School would be a place where Alex could finally become the confident individual she knew he could be.

I fell in love with that family that day. I knew that no matter what, I was going to make sure I did the best I could for Alex, for Dillon, and for all students within that school.

This meeting was a sign from God that I was still passionate about the profession I had chosen, and that my year 28 was going to be just as rewarding as the previous 27 years had been.

I met Marina and her husband another day. Alex was not in attendance. The ARD committee consisted of Alex's home bound teacher, a diagnostician, and the special education teacher that would end up transforming Alex into the confident, capable, and happy young man he is today. Her name is Ms. Amy Snowden.

We all listened as Marina shared stories of concern, of failed programs experienced in other schools, and of cautioned hope in their son's enrollment into the program and Frisco High School. We sat together and made a plan. Little did we know that Alex would not only exceed our wildest expectations, but he would blow us all out of the water with his totally unexpected growth and commitment to being the best Alex, the most popular Alex, he could be.

I learned a long time ago that Special Education is only a title and in no way hinders or limits a child's potential. My own daughter, Meg, is a severe diabetic who was placed under the Special Education umbrella for protection when her diabetes was out of control or she was in the hospital. She graduated high school with a 3.1 GPA and is now a freshman in college. Special Education simply gave her the safety net she needed to excel, even when she was not in the best of health. I knew we had a wonderful student, a plan in place, a great staff, and a shared commitment by family and faculty to help make Alex feel at home and become a successful, happy and confident part of our FHS family.

Throughout the first semester, Alex and I saw each other almost every day. Either I would go and seek him out to say hi or he would find me to let me know he was at school and ready to go. We spoke a lot. We would speak of issues Alex was having with other students and rehearse ways to respond when certain students were unkind. He spent the first half of the day at school and the second half at home with the assistance of a homebound teacher. Marina and Blake called often to check up on Alex and sometimes to ask for advice on how to handle a certain situation. Blake and Marina were always looking out for the best for Alex but increasingly trusting of the input from Amy and me. Amy Snowden and I became more and more confident as the semester wore on that Alex would soon have the ability and desire to become a full time day student. We worked for that. We wanted that.

Right before the winter break, Alex informed me that he had a present for me down in Ms. Amy's room. He said that he just wanted to give his "Aunt Vicki" something for Christmas. It was the most beautiful hand-crafted leather journal I had ever seen. I was so proud and so touched. It was just another symbol of how special Alex, Dillon, and their parents were.

Over the break, Alex took a turn for the worse with the onset of a Bell's Palsy episode that affected his face and one side of his body. When he returned from the holidays, his face was red, his smile constricted, his self esteem squashed. I will never forget the first day I spoke to him after his return. I asked him to show me that smile of his, and he told me he couldn't. It broke my heart. He was so sad. I didn't want to push the conversation since we were in the hall, so I simply told him it would be ok and watched him walk to class, head and eyes to the floor as he walked.

We had a chance to speak in my office a couple of days later. He told me he was sad. He told me he was questioning why all this hardship was placed on him. He told me he just wanted to be normal. As he told me that, I felt a big lump in my throat. I thought to myself, why would you ever want to be normal? No one ever remembers normal! But everyone will always remember Alex. I believe that kids like Alex, and my Meg, were given diseases because they are strong enough to handle it. Alex will be the vehicle by which this disease is further investigated, further researched, and further understood. It is already happening with the publication of his mother's book.

All children are special. All children deserve the best education anyone can give them.

When Marina asked me to contribute to this book, she asked me to speak about how I worked with Alex. My answer, my dear Marina, is that I work with Alex the same way I work with all students. I see all kids as individuals. I see their potential, even if they don't. I help them find their limitations and boundaries, and then I help them break through them. That is what all educators should do. That is what all kids deserve. That is why I still smile driving to work every day.

I have been blessed by knowing the Sharfman family. My life will be forever changed by Alex. I hope that anyone who reads this book will be blessed as well.

Vicki

My name is Amy Snowdon. I am a Special Education teacher but my primary responsibility here at FHS is the SBS room. SBS stand for Specialized Behavior Support. At this time I have 9 students on my case load, including Alex. My responsibilities include helping develop IEP's, behavior goals, giving my particular students a "safe place" to go should they begin to feel overwhelmed and ultimately helping them to be successful in the classroom. I communicate to my students and teachers pertinent information that will help them help the student. In the beginning, Alex used the room quite a bit. We started out having him work in the room with myself or one of my paraprofessionals. His work would be sent to us and we would sit and help him complete it, reading to him for better understanding if we needed too. Since the main objective is to have these students in the classroom and as he became more comfortable, we slowly "weaned" him out of SBS. At first he would go to class for the first half in order to receive the new material and come back to work on assignments. By Christmas, he was in the classroom the whole period, only coming down when he felt he needed support. After the first semester I felt he was doing well enough to stay through third period. Frisco High Schools are on a block schedule so students attend 4 classes a day, alternating "A" days and "B' days. The class periods are 90 minutes long so this was a huge accomplishment for Alex.

The next step was to get him to stay through third period. At our first meeting in August of 2008 when we determined Alex's placement, the ARD committee made sure that these 3rd period classes were not "core "classes (History, Math, Science) The idea was that when and if he made the transition to a longer day it would be less stressful so we enrolled him in some electives – things he would enjoy and look forward to. After the semester started, I checked in with the teachers to see how he was doing. One of them asked me why he was homebound part of the day. When I explained that he had Tourette Syndrome he said he had never noticed the tics and that he handled the class beautifully.

He has come so far and I know it hasn't been easy for him. I'm so proud of what he has accomplished and I can't wait to see what the future holds for him. This experience has given me a new perspective on the saying "it takes a village to raise a child". The staff, teachers and students here are so incredibly open minded and accepting and I know that has contributed to Alex's success.

Amy

TREATMENTS

DISEASE AND DISORDERS/HOW DID WE GET HERE?

Constantine Kotsanis, M.D.

Over the past 200 years the planet Earth and its ecology has seen significant changes due to human disregard of the entire ecosystem. One could argue that technological advances have made life easier and better for everyone, however, the entire perspective of such an individual will change if they have an ASD (Autism Spectrum Disorder) child to raise.

The advances of physics and chemistry have moved our civilization fast-forward over the past two centuries. Knowledge gained, as of this writing, seems to double every two hours and there is no end in sight. Fancy homes and offices, super highways, massive cities, modern transportation systems, and advanced telecommunications, are wonderful for everyone to enjoy and use. However, we have paid a steep toxic price for our luxuries. This is especially true for the parents, families and children of Autism and Tourette Spectrum disorders. Treatment of Tourettes require the following interventions for digestion, gut flora, hyperactivity to allergies, and detoxification.(emptying the toxins from the system).

For example: Alex was brought into my office for a consultation by his parents on October 21st, 2008, to review his family history and discuss a plan to begin treatment. Two weeks later, on November, 3rd, 2009, we began diagnostic testing, including an executive profile, hair analysis for toxic metals, RAST allergy panel, comprehensive stool analysis, plasma amino acids, blood tests for lipids and homocysteine, mineral profile, immune deficiency panel, organic acid profile and phase microscopy.

Alex was a 17 year old male, who eight years prior, had been diagnosed with, Tourette Syndrome. Alex's condition was marked by motor, vocal, and self-injury tics. He had also shown indication of "attention deficit hyper activity disorder, inattentive type, with history of depression and obsessive-compulsive disorder" as stated by his developmental neurologist.

Prior to visiting the Kotsanis Institute, Alex had very little success with medications due to their associated side effects and lack of effectiveness to control his injurious tics. The problem was detrimental to his success in school, as he had to be placed on a limited school-day schedule.

I received Alex's test results on November 24, 2008, showing Alex to have an allergenic reactivity to some foods, imbalance of multiple amino acids, irregularity of his gastrointestinal flora and environmental toxicity. A detailed plan of therapy, including nutrition, supplements, along with future allergy treatment ((LDA) and detoxification were discussed.

The first day of treatment at the Kotsanis Institute began with initial interventions that included a rotation elimination diet as well as supplementation with vitamins, mineral, digestive enzymes and fish oil. Alex was also given vitamin B-12 shots twice a week. On November 26, 2008, I received a phone call from Alex's mother, Marina, reporting that Alex had an increased incidence of tics.I immediately put a plan into action to begin gamma-aminobutyricacid (GABA), along with foot massages with fish oil.

A week later Alex's parents informed me that his tics were not improving and he was experiencing aphthous ulcers in his mouth. A prescription for Kenalog Orabase was called into their pharmacy for his ulcers, along with a prescription for Xyrem (GHB or gamma-hydroxbutric acid) which acts as a sleep aid.

Twenty days later, on December 22nd, 2008, Alex and his parents arrived for his follow- up appointment, declaring that Alex had made a significant progress in all areas, ranging from his overall disposition to his communication, speech, self-injury tics, sleep patterns, bowel habits, and positive interaction with others. They also announced that Alex's tics, in general, had been reduced to the point that they were close to becoming non-existent. They were convinced that the supplements and diet were instrumental in his progress.

On March 3rd, 2009, I had a phone conference with Alex's parents. In little over three and a half months of treatment at the Kotsanis Institute, Alex has shown dramatic improvements in all areas, and according to his parents, had finally become **tic free**.

Prior to the academic year of 2009, Alex was home schooled for four years, due to severe self-injury tics. In 2008 he had threatened to commit suicide on multiple occasions. Academically he was unable to have any passing grades until he started treatment at the Kotsanis Institute. In December of 2008 his outlook had a very significant positive shift in personal and academic achievements. For the first time, his report card exhibited a range from 77 to 92. There is no doubt that the nutritional and gastrointestinal corrections played a major role in Alex's recovery.

I am thrilled to say, that in April, 2009, Alex's high school has reported that he has enough credits to go into his senior year, and has made plans to attend a two year college.

Now that the nutritional interventions have created stability for Alex, I plan to introduce the next two steps of the basic biomedical treatment. This will be LDA (low dose antigen therapy) to control allergy and bring the immune system in line and detoxification to remove all environmental toxins. Most patients have a very favorable response with this approach by the end of the first year of treatment. In summary, using nutrition and drug therapies together as an intervention can be very beneficial, whereas nutrition or drug therapies used alone may not yield the most optimal results.

So what are we dealing with in regards to children like Alex? My first study in 1992 which connected allergies and digestive disorders to autism, came about when I was practicing otolaryngology and allergy ailments. My allergy patients had digestive problems which, if left unattended would keep them from getting control of their allergies. So when a patient was not responding to their allergy shots, the **American Academy of Otolaryngic Allergy** suggested digestive and allergy testing for IgG mediated food allergy biomedical intervention for ASD.

During this time my son was five years old, with all the same allergy and digestive issues as my patients. He also had hyperacusis (overly sensitive hearing). As an ear, nose and throat doctor, when I heard that there was a treatment for hyperacusis (auditory integration training) I bought the equipment for use on my son. The treatment was being used mainly for Autistics and that intrigued me. My son had symptoms of autism that were mild compared to most of the children I considered Autistic, but he was in fact on the **spectrum (a set of additional disorders that are associated with the main disorder).**

My nutritionist and I designed the 1992 autism study to include a record of dietary habits, allowing us to be able to measure nutritional intake. We did comprehensive allergy testing, a comprehensive digestive stool analysis (including parasitology), amino acid and fatty acid testing, immune system panels, and neurotransmitter studies.

In 92% of the cases there were problems with digestion, and in 100% of the cases there were problems with allergies, based on each child's test results, that we treated with antifungals, antiparasitics, antibacterials, probiotics and digestive enzymes. All patients diagnosed with leaky gut syndrome received a preparation combining an amino acid, fatty acid, complex carbohydrate, antioxidant and vitamin E.

My Biomedical treatments for autism spectrum disorders include healing the digestive tract using antifungals and nutrients, eliminating gluten, casein and allergic foods, treating allergies and feeding a nutrient-dense diet. Chelation and other forms of detoxification such as far-infrared saunas are also often necessary. These are the foundation of what has become known as the **"Defeat Autism Now"** or **"DAN"**, interventions.

Additional elements may be added, depending on what progress is made after the basics have been tried. These may include methyl B-12 injections, auditory training, anti-inflammatory treatments and hyperbaric oxygen therapy (HBOT), craniosacral therapy, and prism lenses.

The key to achieving good results from the biomedical treatments is to start them as early as possible, be consistently aggressive, and do them sequentially in the right order. Mothers are the real heroes in this story. In 99% of the families that I have seen, the mother leads the charge in controlling the child's environment and diet, as well as championing the cause with school personnel, family and pediatricians.

Most of the change that has been brought about, regarding the acceptance of these treatments by a larger number of people, has been accomplished by mothers who have educated themselves on biomedical treatments and formed support groups and professional organizations to get the word out.

Autism and the disorders that fall somewhere on this diagnostic band are known as ASD or Autism Spectrum Disorders. This spectrum includes ADD, ADHD, Asperger's, PDD and Tourette's syndrome. Autism is on the severe end of this range while attention deficit, hyperactivity, dyslexia and others are on the milder end. All categories of ASD have increased markedly in the past 20 years with estimates of the number affected ranging from one in 150 to one in 50 and growing in numbers every day.

Environmental Dangers For Your Child's Health

There are many suspected causes but the ones that seem most likely are environmental insults such as chemical and electromagnetic pollution, contaminated immunizations, nutritional deficiencies, metabolic disorders and genetics. When discussing the biomedical treatments known as the **"Defeat Autism Now"** biomedical intervention, it is clear that there is no set protocol, but rather that the treatments are selected based on the metabolic profile of each individual. Even though the vast majority of patients have digestive issues, their testing can look very different, one from the other, and therefore their treatments will also vary. Finding a doctor familiar with biomedical intervention is critical to successfully navigating this path to recovery.

The Autism Spectrum Disorder population has grown in a geometric progression since first labeled in the 1940s. There are many theories about the causes of this syndrome, ranging from environment to genetics. In my long study and clinical observations of this syndrome, I have come to realize that the causes are multi-faceted and the treatments are very complex.

Since 1970 the Autism Spectrum Disorder has grown a disturbing rate. According to many sources, including the worldwide organization, **"Autism Speaks**," the birth rate for autistic children has now reached, 1 out of every 150 children. If this continues, in one to two generations 100 percent of all newborns will have the Autism Spectrum Disorder. *James F. Leckman and Donald J. Cohen, of the Yale Child Study Center, have also voiced concern regarding the growth of the Tourette population. "Tourette Syndrome was considered rare and exotic at one time, (however now,) Tourette Syndrome is a relatively common childhood -onset disorder......"*

The problem has become alarming enough for President Obama to propose the 2010 budget to include $211 million dollars for the "Combating Autism Act" (CAA). In 2006, the CAA authorized $920 million dollars in federal funding over five years to fight autism through biomedical and environmental research, surveillance, awareness and early identification. Although, a recent survey released in the March 2009 issue of **"Pediatrics"**, revealed that fighting autism needs to begin with our primary, and Pediatric segment.

The survey included the perspective of 3,100 physicians, and revealed that many families have expressed frustration with physicians' lack of knowledge about the disorder. Physicians, on the other hand, felt that there was a great need to improve primary care for children with autism and provide education for physicians in how to provide that care.

I believe that in order to improve their primary care one must have a knowledge of the environmental problems that is affecting their mind and body. My clinical observations have revealed that there are also several environmental factors responsible for the mental and physical state of the ASD population.

Chemical Based Products Produce Environmental Pollution

The chemical industry has truly revolutionized modern civilization, but it has also caused irreparable damage to the entire planet. In addition, we have inherited the present mind-set of the food industry that deals with focusing on taste and convenience rather than providing complete nutritional sustenance.

The majority of food available in chain food stores would be hard pressed to qualify for the definition of "fresh." And as popular as organic foods have become, still only a small portion of shelf and produce space is designated for their display because of their low volume in sales, due to their high prices, often two or three times higher than non-organic foods.

Since the majority of families cannot afford to eat organically, foods that have a long shelf life and low prices are used regularly and stored in bulk for hard times. Food companies are geniuses at devising attractive advertisement to give the public the idea that most of their products have a very long shelf life. **But, food with a long shelf life means that most of the nutrients have been stripped and preservatives added.** This makes these foods unfit for human consumption except in areas of famine or war, and should be avoided on a day to day basis.

Therefore, the answer to supplying nutrient filled food to families may be on the shoulders of the government and not the consumer. If the public demands fresh, nutrient filled food that everyone can afford, and the government supports their demand, then the food chains will be forced to start making changes.

There is a popular theory that has been around for about 75 years, that there are four food groups, but scientifically, there are only three food groups: proteins or amino acids; lipids or fats; and carbohydrates, or sugars. Milk has all three food groups in it. If you need to list a fourth food group you could list water and minerals.

An accurate description of food groups should point out if the foods support the immune system (immuno-supportive) or suppress it (immuno-suppressive). All dairy products, with the exceptions of human mother's milk, raw organic milk and organic ghee butter, are immuno-suppressive. Although pasteurization is designed to prevent potential infections from milk consumption, it makes milk immuno-suppressive. For all practical reasons, other than human mother's milk and organic ghee butter, **all milk products should be avoided by the Tourette/Autism Spectrum Disorder population.** Dairy allergies and intolerance are secondary to ingestion of casin, a milk protein.

Be aware that there are three more harmful foods to the ASD population. In the 1940's margarine was invented. Margarine, a synthetic fat, (along with newer synthetic fats) is primarily responsible for most food related chronic illness proliferation. Fats are the key to good health. The second, synthetic sugars, have been used in great quantities since 1960s and are responsible for many ailments.

The third is the ***genetically modified organism*** (GMO) foods. Very few consumers have any idea how animals and plants are genetically modified, or why. The food chemical industry will argue that they are trying to feed the growing needs of an explosive population. This is true. Although GMO foods will serve the starving populations of the world, they offer no benefit to the individual with Autism Spectrum Disorder. In general, GMO foods are immuno-suppressive.

I have seen, firsthand, the benefit of whole organic food, therefore, bringing me to the conclusion that in my professional opinion the food industry should concentrate on growing safe foods for the entire population, especially children with mental and physical disorders. The future of the world depends on the availability of organic, non toxic food, free of chemicals, antibiotics, hormones, synthetic fats, sugars, and genetically modified foods.

The **Natural Solutions Foundation** has reported that virtually all transgenic (GMO) crops originate in the U.S. As of this writing, the FDA and USDA are still operating under a 1992 Executive Order which states that modified and unmodified foods are equivalent. Therefore, no safety or other testing is required and both FDA and the USDA refuse to require or examine safety testing. The only thing that is required to release a food into the food chain and environment is to obtain a patent.

The third problem faced by the Tourette/Autism Spectrum Disorder population, as well as the general public, is the pharmaceutical industry. The 20th century will be remembered as the golden era of antibiotics. Since the invention of penicillin there has been a bonanza of life saving antibiotics. However, this group of great drugs no longer holds the same effectiveness as it once held, and for some children and adults, many of these medicinal warriors have become totally ineffective because of the overuse of prescriptions by doctors, and the food industry. Unfortunately, we can do little about our doctor's position on antibiotics, but we can speak-out for change in what the food industry is forcing us to eat.

The **"Organic Consumers Association"** published an article by The Washington Post staff, Marc Kaufman, regarding the dangers we face because of the antibiotics that are being mixed into livestock feed by the farmers. According to Mr. Kaufman's findings, the daily or monthly feeding of antibiotics into the livestock causes microbes in the animals to become resistant to the drugs. The consumer can then become infected with the resistant bacteria by eating or handling meat contaminated with the pathogens.

In 1928 Alexander Fleming discovered penicillin. One year later he warned us that bacteria had already managed to devise its own way of surviving the drug. The pharmaceutical industry ignored Flemings's concerns and went on a multibillion dollar selling spree for the next 70 years. Only recently have the pharmaceutical companies understood Fleming's concerns, now they are slowly opting out of costly, major antibiotic research.

However, the food industry continues to use more than 90 percent of the total antibiotics on the market for animal feed. This long term practice is either done out of ignorance or greed, ignoring the bacterial facts of the effects on the livestock and the consumer, brings a harvest of disaster upon us.

The ability of the micro kingdom to figure out new threats and learn to cope with them makes them superior to any form of life this Earth has ever seen. Testimony to this fact is that they are the only species that have survived all assaults of nature and catastrophic event, ever since they appeared on this planet about 3.8 billion years ago. Their keen ability to mutate and share information with other forms of life makes them the ultimate survivors.

Within 100,000 bacterial lifetimes the micro kingdom rendered antibiotics practically useless in less than 75 years from their discovery. Thus, I believe scientists are forced to cooperate with the ecosystem or threaten extinction of humans. Last, but not least, the food industry must stop using antibiotics in the food chain. Failure to do so will certainly result in a severe impairment of humans by the micro kingdom and the ecosystem in general.

Remember that the primary function of the micro kingdom is to keep the ecosystem free of garbage and parasitic activities. For the past 200 years humans have behaved like parasites against the ecosystem. The micro kingdom is only doing what it is genetically programmed to do.

The basic facts and laws of nature cannot be disputed. We must remember that the laws of nature should be utilized by humans for the express purpose of promoting balance between all living and non-living components of the ecosystem. It is time for the scientific community to realize they cannot bend the laws of nature. It is time for the scientific community to realize "pure science" cannot save us from intellectual arrogance, and gross disregard of the ecosystem. It will take political and true scientific resolve to return the planet Earth to its original intended form and purpose. The discipline of science demands verifiable evidence by everyone who seeks the truth. Political correctness, fiscal convenience, exploitation of people and natural resources have no place in medicine and science.

During my residency I was able to completely comprehend and embrace the great American Medical Association training, along with the thought process to which it was partnered. I was convinced, up to the first five post graduate years of my long career, that the AMA was only a step below God. This feeling of AMA divinity sharply came to an end when I discovered that my son was on the Autism Spectrum, during my formal medical training. When I started looking for answers for my son, I ran into the AMA brick wall. Just like most parents with ASD children, I was ridiculed when I tried to make any connections between the rapid demise of his health to vaccinations.

A lengthy literature search shows very little is written about the maturity of the immune system. The literature available shows that the immune system reaches maturity between the ages of 2 to 4 years of age. Furthermore, the literature shows that the child does not reach significant immune competency until about the age of 2 years. Thus, it would be difficult to develop an antigen-antibody complex (the intended purpose of vaccination) in the first two years of life.

To develop an antibody-antigen reaction is a prerequisite one needs for an intact immune system. Children are immuneo-compromised under the age of 2 years because their immune system has not yet completely developed. Traditional literature also documents that 20 percent of all premature babies are immuneo-compromised. Yet I have not seen a single article in any discipline warning parents of the dangerous practice of childhood vaccinations for the premature infant.

When I was growing up as a child, we did not receive vaccinations until we entered the first grade. My generation has done very well with minimal vaccinations at the appropriate age. Humanity is now in peril due to over-vaccinating the population-especially in a compressed time schedule. In my clinical experience with health and disease in this population, minimal vaccinations should be offered to immuno-compromised individuals, only after their immune system has matured. I believe that the new standard of care should include that a physician must test his/her patient for immuno-competency prior to any vaccinations.

ASD has long been linked to genetic and familial predispositions, creating major guilt among parents. If a child is diagnosed with Autism Spectrum Disorder, there is a 33 percent chance that a second sibling will also develop ASD. Of all premature births, 20 percent are immuno-compromised and 2 to 5 percent of all births carry genetic mutations. This might leave one to surmise that all diseases are connected to compromised genes of genetic origin. However, it would be wise to look closer by exploring toxic foods and toxic environments in order to discover the reason for compromised genetic expression.

If the environment could be restored to its original format, most, if not all, genetically implicated diseases would self-correct. Historically, if you were to study toxicity in human bones before and after the "Industrial Revolution" you would find about a 2,500 percent increase in toxins compared to humans living before the "Industrial Revolution." It is apparent that toxicity and not genetics is the underlining cause of ASD, as well as most diseases of the 21st Century.

The steps to health require removal of toxic foods, toxic drugs and toxic thoughts. The only way out of the "post industrial revolution civilization disease" is to go back to the drawing board and rethink what we are doing to each other and the ecosystem in general. For the industrialists and the scientific community, this is a golden opportunity to take the planet Earth to the next level of prosperity, and move humanity out of the dark ages of reckless disrespect and dogmatic teachings against the ecosystem.

I am looking forward to the day that the leaders in Washington, and the UN, will place humanity and planet Earth ahead of ego and greed. We need a change of attitude in the way we treat the ecosystem. Failure to do so will most certainly mark the end of human occupation of planet Earth before the turn of the next century.

Let's all wake up to the greatest possession God has given to humanity, i.e., "love and compassion" toward one another, and all living and non living things of the planet Earth.

Homeopathy

Treating The Whole Person
Rhonda Majalca D.H. CHom

Homeopathy is a holistic system of treatment developed by Dr. Samuel Hahnemann in the 1800's. His first findings were based on experimenting on himself. He ingested Peruvian bark containing quinine; when he developed the same symptoms as malaria, he successfully used the quinine to cure the malaria in his patients. More than 200 years later, classical homeopaths have continued to use his scientific rules to this day.

Why did Dr. Hahemann make himself sick? For the same reasons people seek out homeopathic remedies today. He believed that the strong drugs being consumed at that time did more harm than good. He was looking for a natural alternative. In addition to severe side effects, traditional medicine also has a much higher price tag, and it subscribes to the concept that "one size fits all" in treating patients with similar symptoms.

The origin of the name Homeopathy comes from two Greek words that mean "like disease." The concept behind homeopathy is that natural substances have the healing power to cure illnesses with the very symptoms that they are known for. Think about the natural healing powers of the red onion, for instance. The juice of a red onion can cause us to have red and watery eyes, while a dilution of allium cepa (red onion) is used to treat watery, burning eyes. Like cures like.

The idea of like-cures-like is not limited to homeopathic medicine. Modern day allergy treatments work in much the same way. The patient is exposed to the allergen in order to increase their tolerance to the allergy. Similarly, consider the finding of Louis Pasteur. He discovered vaccines by injecting a form of the disease in a healthy person in an attempt to fend off the disease. This is also the premise of the seasonal flu shot

How Does Homeopathy Differ From Traditional Medicine?

In order to effectively treat a patient, Dr. Hahnemann believed that the practitioner has to do more than just look at the physical symptoms. This is literally what a "holistic" approach means. Homeopathic practitioners take into consideration the present state of the patient's mind and body before determining the appropriate remedy. When our **"being"** is out of balance and unhealthy, it is believed that our body alerts us through physical symptoms. Our bodies are designed to be in balance with our emotional and mental needs as well.

Consider twin siblings who are both experiencing migraine headaches, but because of other factors in their lives, their homeopathic remedies may be completely different. Each patient has a different lifestyle (stress level), different dietary habits as well as different personality traits. In this example the exact same remedy will not necessarily work in both of the patients.

Does Homeopathy Work for Both Acute and Chronic Illness?

Homeopathy has been successful in reducing and eliminating the symptoms of many illnesses, both acute and chronic.

Acute Condition: Any condition that lasts one day or less than two weeks and is self limiting (cold, flu, ear ache, rash, bruise, etc. A brief 10 to 25 minute consultation is needed to help address your current condition. Acute conditions can be taken care of by the client or the practitioner, depending on your preference. You should keep track of the remedies you use and why you used them.

Chronic Condition: Any condition that you have had for more than two or more weeks (allergies, sinus, PMS, menopause, arthritis, etc.) or if you have seen a medical doctor and are on medication. For chronic conditions it is best to visit a professional homeopath for an in-depth assessment, a one hour to two hour consultation addressing your current health care concerns.

What Happens During A Consultation?

"It is more important to know what sort of person has a disease than to know what sort of disease a person has." -Hippocrates

A consultation with a homeopath is like meeting someone for the first time and they want to get to know all about you. You will have the luxury of spending two hours to talk about yourself, your needs, wants, aches, pains, what makes you happy, sad, anxious or angry. And this will be a completely different experience for you as not one will be interrupting you and telling their own similar stories or simply responding with "How does that make you feel."

Your homeopath will review your case for a day of two. If she/he feels the need to have more information, the homeopath will call you and get clarification before recommending a remedy.

A review of your case is very important. Everything that was discussed will be reviewed and key words in your case will help to find a remedy for you. The more open you are during your consultation the deeper the remedy will help in the body.

Your Remedy!

Your individual remedy has the ability to stimulate your body's own healing progression; because it works in conjunction with your body's natural curative process, it is very important to take the remedy as recommended by your homeopath. Your condition and how sensitive your system is will determine how much and how often to take the remedy. Some patients will only take a dose one time in three months. Another person might have to take a dose three times a day, everyday. You will be given written instructions on how to take the remedy, which will help you understand how much and how often you will take the remedy.

Ask your doctor's advice if you plan on discontinuing your prescription medication. It is important for your doctor to monitor you during that time. Also inform your doctor that you are working with a homeopath and you have taken a homeopathic remedy.

Once you begin the process you may not need to re-dose for two to three months, or you might have to dose more often. That is one of the reasons why the follow-ups are important. The second reason is to decide whether the remedy given to you in the beginning is still working for you or if a change is necessary. Lastly, we determine if the potency is working for you.

The healing process is different for everyone depending on the length of time the individual has had their condition. A few days, weeks, a year, or many years, because each person is unique in the way they experience their disease, they will heal in their own way and time. The body cannot be rushed in the healing process. Not even a cut on the finger goes away fast enough for us. I have seen remedies work in less than five minutes to taking six months, a year and sometimes longer.

What is it that each of us gains by having our condition? This is really hard for some people to realize. They may have fears about getting better. Maybe their friends and family won't spend as much time with them. They won't be the center of everyone's attention anymore. Then there is the case of people who are in a hurry to get well. For them, it can't happen fast enough. But are they really ready for it. Changes that happen too fast will cause even more stress. It's new to them.

Constant stress is top of the chart for most people. Some medication can and will work against remedies, negating the benefits of a good remedy. That is why it is important to let your homeopath know all of the medications you are taking in the present and what you have taken in the past. Be sure to inform your doctors that you are working with a professional homeopath.

Reactions differ among individuals, because a homeopath is working with the whole body, the mental, emotional, and the physical aspect. When a person is given a remedy, until the client comes in for a follow up we won't know how deep the remedy has reached. Homeopaths want to reach the deepest part of the mental/emotional body; once that has been achieved the physical complaint will start to resolve itself. Because of the chemical make-up in everyone, each person is unique, and this is why the homeopath doesn't give the same remedy to two or more people with the same condition. We try to find the strange, rare, and peculiar symptoms the individual is experiencing, not just the common symptoms for that complaint.

Healing The Family As A Unit
Children With Mental/Behavior Disorders

Parents that are caring for children with behavior disorders do not realize that their children will react to the parents' stress and suffering. If the parents are stressed, the child will pick up on it and react in the best (or worst) way they know, at home and at school. Over a long period of time this can add to the child's problem with family and the whole community. We are all connected and all of us need to be part of the healing process.

We have heard of families falling apart, or one person in the family on a mission to help the child that is stressed to the point of their health being affected. Parents have to remember that they have to take care of themselves first, in order to be able to care for their children. The more you take the time to care for yourself, the better you can take care of your child. A parent that is stressed out, not getting the rest they need, will only fall apart, burn out, or end up in the hospital.

It is crucial for the family to seek homeopathic care. If a child member is suffering from disorders such as ADHD, OCD, Tourette, Bi-polar, etc., it is affecting the whole family, not just the child. In fact,it is affecting the community in which the child lives. When helping the whole family, everyone is receiving the help they need to eliminate stress. Things just seem to work out better for the family without everyone realizing that it's happening. Sort of like a light bulb going on. Mothers find they are not as stressed and life seems to be less complicated. Soon they come out of their mental fog and can focus on what they need and want to do.

What Happens When My Child Is Healed?

When a child has had a long difficult disorder and is finally healed, there may be years of past pain and trauma that the parent may wonder how that will affect the child's future. All we can do is work from this point forward. Our past defines who we are as a person, and how we respond to people and circumstances in our life.

A child that has gone through a chronic situation just wants to be treated as normal. What is normal to them is very important. When they say, "I just want to be normal," ask your child what they think would make them feel normal. You might be surprised. The following definitions are just a few of the the answers I have received as a professional:

1. "Normal for me is to be treated like my brothers/sisters. I don't want to be treated different. I feel guilty because my parents spend so much time with me at the hospital. They yell at my siblings and it's not always their fault."

2. "Normal to me would not to feel invisible. I just want my parents to notice me."

3. "Normal to me would be to be treated like everyone else, with respect."

4. "Normal for me would be having a girl friend like all the other guys in school."

6. "Normal for me is being able to have a driver's license."

7. "Normal to me would be to have everyone listen to what I have to say, like you do, without passing judgement or making comments."

8. "Normal for me would be for people not to look at me like I was a freak."

I believe that the idea of "being normal" is a delusion of what we see in others that we would like to see in ourselves. This is why listening to your children's feelings is so important. If they feel good about themselves, they will make better decisions, at home and at school, making them better prepared to handle the physical aspect of their lives.

When a child thinks that no one understands them everything they think and do is fear based. Fear can be very detrimental to a person by keeping them from doing the things they love in life. Fear can make a person freeze when they are in a life or death situation. Sadly, fear can bring some people to take their own life or the lives of others.

Homeopathy helps to tap into the spiritual side of us. Once we start taking remedies our hearts begin to open the possibilities of a better life and a peace come over us that effects us on all levels. The phrase, "stop, observe and listen," comes to mind. Stop what you are doing, observe your child without comment. Listen to the words your child is speaking; this is their truth. This is how they see the world.

Remember when we used to say, "sticks and stones can break our bones?" Well, those bones will heal and the pain will be forgotten, but the lack of caring words, can hurt deep inside of a child for the remainder of their life. Love your children, make them feel unique in every way, and don't let their disorder or disease define who they are. Be the instrument of God by instilling peace and joy into their life.

––––––––––

Rhonda Majalca D.H., CHom received her diploma and certification from the Homeopathic Academy of Southern California. She is a Registered Bio Energetic Technician since 2001 and attained the highest award for her training at the American Institute of Energy Medicine. She has been involved in the medical community for more than 15 years working with renowned doctors and their patients both in traditional and alternative medicine.

Her interest in investigating the causal factors of disease led to her attainment and proficiency in Homotoxicology from the International Society of Homotoxicology.

She is available for lectures and is a member of the Chula Vista Chamber of Commerce, San Diego Chamber of Commerce, BBB Accredited business, National Center for Homeopathy, North American Society of Homeopaths. In addition, she facilitates a monthly NCH affiliated study Group; hosts a domestic violence support group at her church, and is on the auxiliary for Project Safe House.

––––––––––

INDIGENOUS APPROACHES TO HEALING WITH SPECIAL REFERENCE TO AUTISM

By Barbara Mainguy, MFA and Lewis Mehl-Madrona, MD,PhD, MPhil
Concordia University, Montreal, Argosy University Hawai'i, and University of Hawai'i at Manoa

Within the indigenous worldview, all healing is fundamentally spiritual healing. All of the indigenous healers with whom we studied or collaborated relied on spirits as the source of all inspiration for healing. Spirits were everywhere. Within indigenous healing systems, supernatural beings guide the treatment. Indigenous healing here involves dancing, drumming, rattling and singing, in a non invasive manner in which even autistic children can engage. Elders are adept at narratives without words. The sacred songs of ceremonies convey rich cultural messages through music. Elders teach people diagnosed with autism to participate in their specific socio-cultural context through whole body communication. Rather than teaching a set of behaviors the elders encourage increased self-awareness/self-other awareness, leading to more overt social interactions.

A recent area of interest is the shared ideology (and perhaps shared roots) between aboriginal healing concerns and modern day creative arts therapies, which are often used with children with autism. Music therapy principles can link to what elders do with the children and can also play an important role for parents of children with autism by fostering relationships and developing positive interactions. Most approaches to music therapy rely on spontaneous musical improvisation just as elders do. Drumming also has its impact as musical therapy. Dance movement therapy and drama therapy are also used with autistic children: Body centered therapies can bring important comfort to individuals struggling with autism and parallel the spontaneous cultural therapies into which elders introduce autistic individuals.

To the surprise of biomedical trained practitioners, most indigenous healing systems conceptualize illness very differently.sdfootnote2sym Contemporary medicine bases its diagnoses on structural changes in tissues, while indigenous cultures are more concerned with disharmony and imbalances in social relationships (Mehl-Madrona, 2003). Medicine is noun based, while indigenous thought is verb based. While biomedicine traces the sources of structural tissue changes, indigenous healers contemplate the source for disturbances in the harmony of individuals within their communities and in all their relationships. When the harmony within relationships is disturbed, imbalances result that lead to illness and therefore to suffering. The two views are not necessarily contradictory. They can be linked, though not within the restricted perspective of contemporary biomedicine. The linkage occurs from our observation that sufficient degrees of disharmony and imbalance lead to tissue damage. It is associated with suffering. For example, different cytokines (messenger molecules of inflammation) are out of balance for a variety of disease (arthritis, asthma, diabetes). Different imbalances are seen for each disease; what is consistent is the presence of imbalance.

The "natural history of disease" concept of biomedicine compares and contrasts to one of disharmony and imbalance in which larger levels of disharmony are associated with greater strength for those forces that oppose health. To accept this, we must accept the idea that how we live and the stories we enact, relate to the health of our bodies and that our psychological resilience parallels, in some manner, our physical resilience. Biomedicine has difficulty traveling here though the concept is becoming more commonly discussed in narrative medicine circles (Mehl-Madrona, 2007).

Indigenous healing is usually viewed through a narrow, non-historical lens by biomedicine, which is convinced of its own supremacy and correctness regardless of the era. This is despite recommendations and beliefs about the causes of disease and the best treatments changing frequently. When we change our thinking in medicine, we behave as if we have always thought in our new way. Treatments do change with regularity, and we promptly forget the treatments in which we previously believed, acting as if whatever we believe today was always true, and we always believed it. A good example of this comes from comments by Mooney published in 1856 who wrote that the Cherokee stuck porcupine quills and thorns into people as treatment for illness when every civilized person knew that the proper treatment was to bleed with leeches. The Cherokee were practicing acupuncture, having had a long established tradition of appreciation of energy meridians and of the value in needling areas of blockage. The attitude of biomedicine toward indigenous healing has changed little since 1856, though we are no longer bleeding people with leeches and have embraced to some extent acupuncture. Stainless steel, sterile needles are used by both physicians and Cherokee healers nowadays, because they are available and work better. Indigenous healers tend to appropriate elements from around them when it is clear that these tools or techniques have merit, and stainless steel needles are no exception.

Spirits and spiritual healing. What separates biomedicine most from contemporary indigenous healing is the belief in spirits and their role in healing, though we have heard it argued at anthropology conferences, that medicine's almost blind faith in pharmaceuticals over all other therapies almost constitutes a religion. For medicine, science has eliminated all supernatural practices and influences, though small departments and centers of spirituality and health attempt to reawaken our sense of the importance of its importance. Within the indigenous worldview, all healing is fundamentally spiritual healing. Even plants heal through the transfer of the spirit of the plant and its spiritual energy into the person ingesting the plant, requiring a sacred preparation of the plants that are to be given.

All of the indigenous healers with whom I studied or collaborated relied on spirits for healing. Spirits were real to them. They talked to spirits daily – natural spirits such as the spirit of the lake by which he or she lived, the spirit of a river, the spirit of the medicinal plants with whom he or she worked, and, of course, departed relatives and healers who assisted in the curing process. Without these many relationships, the healer could not function. Spirits guided their diagnosis of the disharmony and imbalance through dreams and visions and speaking in ceremonies. Spirits entered into the body of the sick person to do curing. Spirits were everywhere.

This magical worldview makes the universe seem friendlier and more agreeable. It places us as relatively minor beings in a universe of consciousness, aspects of it being vast. I didn't see any contradiction between science and talking to spirits, though this is perhaps not the most common view. I described my upbringing by Cherokee grandparents in *Coyote Medicine* (Mehl-Madrona, 1998), in which I described the matter of fact way in which healers related to spirits, interacted with them, and accepted their help. However, they were not dogmatic. If biomedicine could offer help, they would accept it. However, my grandmother's perspective was that spirits were more reliable, though she did take medications to heal her pulmonary tuberculosis and was glad that they existed. She was not prejudiced against anything that worked. One of my relatives said, "If it works, it's good medicine."

A difference comes in our judging whether or not "it works" by our own eyes and not through blind faith in the results of randomized, controlled trials as recommended by evidence-based medicine. Our perspective is more outcome-based. Science is the systematic observation, description, and analysis of relationships and their effects. Indigenous healing has its own kind of science in which healers studiously assess their results for their reputation hinges on their percent of successes over failures. We can also systematically assess the outcomes of healers and compare these outcomes to similar patients seen by biomedical practitioners or add healers to patients who have achieved maximal benefit from biomedicine. Healers must be able to use all their tools. None would see the demands of an RCT as ethical – that is, doing just one intervention the same way for everyone. They could not function that way, for the spirits never give them the same instructions twice. Every person who consults them is unique and receives a unique set of instructions and unique treatments and ceremonies.

Within indigenous healing systems, supernatural beings guide the treatment. Spirits tell the healer what to do as opposed to a rational system in which logic determines action. This comes as frustration to biomedically trained practitioners who want to know how indigenous healers treat "arthritis." One elder answered this question by saying, "I don't know Arthritis. Bring her around tomorrow and I will get to know her and I will let you know what I could do for her." His tongue was in his cheek as he said this, but he made his point. He didn't have a treatment algorithm for arthritis as the biomedical practitioner did. He had to consult the spirits in every instance and develop a unique treatment plan for every person based upon their individual and family and cultural needs.

In most indigenous contexts, treatments match people instead of the biomedical diagnosis. Other constructs exist for causality including breaking taboos, being cursed, and, primarily, being in the midst of relationship disturbances on any level, including social, natural, and spiritual. For any problem, the healer approaches the person instead of the symptoms, asking "Where is your specific disharmony or imbalance." For example, when I injured my knee and could hardly walk, my elder, John C., never touched it. Instead, John prayed and dreamed and determined from his dreams that I had been cursed. He described the person who was cursing me, whom Lewis recognized. Then we prayed for her and he prayed for me. He covered me with a sheet and burned herbs under the sheet until I thought he was going to run out of air. He fanned me with his eagle wing and sang and prayed further. Then he gave me "medicine" (a pouch containing herbs tied to eagle feathers and ribbons) to hang on his truck's mirror to reflect back the curse. I immediately felt much better. One week later John "doctored" me again and gave him"medicine" to put on my front door. My knee was completely better one week later.

John C. did not have to touch my knee to know what was wrong. His dreams told him. Perhaps he intuited the dynamics involved. Perhaps spirits told him.

The indigenous concept of people who are sick accepts the uncertainty of ever having an explanation. Perhaps only spirits could know the reasons for illness. Perhaps entreaty to the spirits could improve the condition; perhaps, not. But treatment planning requires spirit input. Spirits are asked what to do and how to proceed. Next the healer aims to restore harmony and balance to a disturbed situation. The healers work with whatever is presented, not knowing what is possible, but trusting that engaging the spirits in a dialogue could start a healing process.

Examples from autistic spectrum disorders. In a separate paper, I (Mehl-Madrona, ms. under editorial review, 2009) reported upon the beneficial effects of traditional healers for children who had received autistic spectrum diagnoses. The elders were effective as exemplified in some illustrative cases. In the next section, we will discuss potential explanations for this efficacy.

Case 1. Michael was a 23-year-old adult who had been diagnosed with moderately severe autism. Michael had lived most of his life in Winnipeg, but had recently been brought back to his home reserve in Saskatchewan because his mother feared for her own health and wanted Michael to develop relationships with other relatives to sustain him in the event that she became too ill to care for him or died.

When Michael first arrived he showed minimal interest in any social relationships. His interest was playing music on the rims of water glasses, which he did for hours, as well as flushing toilets to see the water spin down (also for long periods of time), and collecting match box cars. He also talked incessantly about lizards. When the traditional healer met him, the healer played water glass music also, watched the toilet water flush with him, and gifted him with a new match box car. The healer brought one more implement – a drum. While they were doing other activities, the healer began to drum… and drum … and drum. Eventually Michael was engrossed in the drumming, nodding his head in rhythm. Finally the healer handed Michael the drum and invited him to play. Almost magically another drum appeared and they banged away together.

I know that Michael's mother had given the healer tobacco in request for his help with Michael, but could afford little else. She had barely enough money to stay stocked with cigarettes. The healer clearly cared about Michael as did others in the community. He kept coming to visit Michael. Slowly but surely they developed a relationship focused upon the drums. Subtly the elder began to add singing and chanting to the drumming. Michael began humming along. Over time he began to learn the words. The elder sat with him periodically. The elder also gave Michael a can of paint and let him paint anything he wished on the elder's house. Michael spent hours on this project in which the elder joined him occasionally, painting along with him or chatting away.

Eventually Michael began attending ceremonies. He appeared very proud to be within the Inipi, to be drumming. The elder gave him a special sweat drum to bring to ceremony. Michael was beginning to form social awareness. Over the course of the next four years, Michael became progressively more oriented into the healer's "hocokah," or circle of people who relied upon him. Then his mother died. Michael cried, but virtually the entire community came out for him. The funeral lasted four days as was customary. Michael was seamlessly integrated into the community. He danced at powwows. Over four years, Michael had developed more of a social self.

Case 2. Donald was a 3 year old child diagnosed with autism. Consistent with contemporary Canadian health care, Donald had waited 18 months from recognition to diagnosis. No services were available to him once diagnosed. Donald lived on a reserve about 2 hours north of Saskatoon. Friends of Donald's mother encouraged her to connect with me. My first response, despite whatever else could be done, was to introduce Donald and his mother to one of their local healers. (This was a huge part of my work in Saskatchewan.) I encouraged Faye, Donald's mother, to start coming to ceremony and bringing Donald. Donald was initially relatively new to human contact. This example convinced me that community could overcome great obstacles. We watched Donald make great strides to catch up with his age-mates. More than just the drumming and singing and dancing, Donald became a most adorable pow-wow dancer, even when he was clueless about how to dance. His mom learned to make elaborate costumes, which made up for his missed steps and puzzled expressions on his face.

More than the support for Donald, was the support for his single mother. People often underestimate the support that a community can provide, despite poverty and adverse conditions. Faye had previously run in a hard group – drugs, heavy drinking, and gangsters. The shock of Donald's diagnosis opened a door in her heart to embrace the traditional stories of her Cree origins. She sat for long talks with elders. She began learning traditional ways. Three years later, when I had to leave Canada, Donald was dramatically improved.

Case 3. Ralph was 8 years old and insisted on dressing like a rabbit. He wouldn't go outside without his bunny ears. He liked wearing bunny shoes as well. Ralph liked to watch fire. He lit matches whenever possible and stared at the flame until the fire burned his fingers. His parents lived in fear that he would burn down the house. He communicated very little except through lighting fires.

Ralph couldn't sit unless he was wearing his bunny ears and his bunny shoes. Otherwise, he would pace incessantly. If enough time elapsed without his bunny slippers, he would begin to bang his head against the wall.

When Ralph's family moved back to the reserve (because a house opened in which they could live), Ralph was slowly adopted by the community. At first people were scared of him. With time, he grew on everyone. The elder began to invite him to light the fire to heat the stones for the sweat lodge ceremony. Others let him burn their garbage. Others protected him when he ventured into dangerous places on the reserve and kept him from hurting himself. Eventually Ralph had free run of the entire reserve, because everyone took care of him.

Over time, Ralph became interested in the pipe. I suppose it was because it kept being lit on fire. Here is a story the elder told this autistic boy about his sacred pipe:

Long ago, when the world was new and empty, a tribe of people came to live on the lands which are now around The Blue Mountains. At this time, the animals still talked to people, often without words, teaching them how to survive and how to care for the land. These original, almost see-through people were called the One True People. A brave and battle-proven warrior woman called Arrow Woman lived in this tribe...

Arrow Woman was adept with the bow, the spear and the knife. Arrow Woman could shoot straighter with the bow than anyone. She could throw split a branch no bigger than your thumb with a thrown knife, and she could silently throw the spear into eye of a hawk in flight.

One day while on a hunt, Arrow Woman came upon the paw prints of Yona the bear. She saw a trail of blood drops upon the ground and knew him to be wounded so she followed his tracks. High above the clouds and into the mountains she followed. Eventually she came to a place of mist and fog that she did not recognize. In this place known only to the animals, she finally saw Yona the bear. He had a deep cut in his side and was bowed down in prayer toward a field of tall grass. The wind swirled around him as he spoke an unknown language. Abruptly, the grass shimmered, almost explosively, and became a lake.

Yona dove into the water. After a time he emerged and his side was completely healed. Yona then saw Arrow Woman and walked to her. Yona told her, "this is the sacred lake of the animals. Its location is known only to the animals. It is where we come for healing and strength. You are the first human to have ever seen the sacred lake.

"You must never tell your kind of its location for it is the home of The Great Uktena." With these words Yona the Bear turned and walked into the woods and disappeared.

Arrow Woman was tired after following Yona all day so she decided to rest a while by this lake. She built a small fire and sat down to the food she had brought. She took a drink of water from the shimmering, silvery lake and felt instantly refreshed. She was amazed to feel as strong as Yan'si the Buffalo. She felt as if she run faster than Coga the Raven could fly.

The woods were quiet, The sun was bright. Unole, the wind, was sleeping. The moon sat low on the horizon, ready to disappear. The surface of the lake was completely calm. At the moment in which Arrow Woman began to get sleepy, she saw Uktena. She had heard of him when she was a child but no one in her tribe ever claimed to have seen him. High above the water he raised his great serpent's head, the jewel in his forehead glistening.

He began to move toward her. Arrow Woman grabbed up her spear and stood proud to face the great creature, showing no fear, the way any warrior should. She raised her spear and prepared to strike the huge beast.

Uktena stopped a short distance from her. He smiled, and his mouth was larger than a man was tall and full of teeth longer than man's forearm. He spoke to the brave woman on the bank of his lake. He said, "Put down your weapons for I mean you no harm. I come only to teach." Arrow Woman laid down her spear and began to relax, her body feeling the truth in Uktena's speech.

He told her to sit and to listen. He dipped his head below the surface and came back up a moment later, holding a strangely crooked stick in his mouth and carrying a leather pouch. He laid these things on the ground in front of Arrow Woman. Then he began to teach, saying, "This that I have laid before you is the Sacred Pipe of The Creator." He told her to pick up the pipe. "The bowl is of the same red clay The Creator used to make human beings. The red clay is for women and is from the Earth. Just as a woman bears the children and brings forth life, the bowl bears the sacred tobacco (tsula) and brings forth smoke. The stem is Man, rigid and strong from the plant kingdom. It supports the bowl just as man supports his family."

Uktena then showed Arrow Woman how to join the bowl to the stem saying, "Just as a man and a woman remain separate until joined in marriage so too are the bowl and stem separate. Never join them unless the pipe is to be used." Uktena then showed her how to place the sacred tsula into the pipe and with an ember from the fire lit the tsula so it burned slightly. He said, "The smoke is the breath of The Creator. When you draw the smoke into your body, you will be cleansed and made whole. When the smoke leaves your mouth, it will rise to The Creator. Your prayers, your dreams, your hopes and desires will be taken to Him in the smoke. Also the truth in your soul will be shown to Him when you smoke the pipe. If you are not true, do not smoke the pipe. If your spirit is bad and you seek to deceive, do not smoke the pipe."

Uktena continued his lesson well into the darkest of nights, sharing all of the prayers used with the pipe and all of the reasons for using the pipe. He finished just as the moon was beginning her bright, nightly journey across the sky in search of her true love. He told Arrow Woman to wrap the pipe in cloth, keeping the parts separate. With this done He told her that she would never again be able to find this place but to remember all that she had learned. Uktena then returned to depths of the lake. Arrow Woman saw the water shimmer phosphorescent and become again the field of grass. She left, taking with her the red stone pipe and her lessons and a wondrous tale. Ever since that time, The People have used the sacred pipe and never again has any man seen the sacred lake of Uktena.

Ralph seemed to listen to the elder's stories indirectly. He slowed his play, attending longer to a particular object, and returned to his former speed and easy distractibility only after the story ended. Over time, Ralph began to act as if he were more aware of the elder. He slowly developed a sense of social relatedness though it took 4 years for him to have a conversation with the elder. By eight years Ralph was interacting almost normally. He seemed to respond to the containment by the community, to the persistent efforts of the elder to engage him, to the music, the rhythm, the consistency of humans in his life, and to the presence of his family.

Explanation. The dancing, drumming, rattling and singing, involved in Indigenous healing is non-invasive, such that even Autistic children can engage and healing can begin. The interaction through music and other non-verbal means becomes a foundation for verbal narratives. These narratives or stories play a near-universal role in the construction of identity and culture among indigenous people (King, 2003). Stories are a means of communication, of retaining history, and of teaching. They are a fundamental way of informing others about culture. Stories always contain a message. The non-verbal stories in which the elder engaged the autistic children slowly led to verbal stories, all embedded in the cultural context found upon the reserve. These stories all emphasize feeling connected, an interrelatedness that extends to the entire universe as a foundational belief of indigenous people (Lux, 2004).

Autism is defined as difficulties in social relationships and those resulting skills that are formed by social relationships, language being primary. Cultural competency (which children diagnosed with autism lack) may depend upon the child's understanding and speaking words sufficient to participate in conversational negotiations with other people about the infinite details of life that require the cooperation of others (Gratier & Trevarthen, 2008). Perhaps children who are diagnosed as autistic (or autistic spectrum) are relatively compromised in the capacity of infants to engage in what Trevarthen (1990, 1994) calls a "non-verbal semiosis of mimetic expression and sympathetic action". He (1974) and Bateson (1979) note that infants show a precocious sense of rhythm and an interest in the qualities, of intention and interest in their mothers' sounds. Reddy (2008) believes that infants begin to sense feelings and purposeful sites of mind in others through lively non-verbal exchanges involving both vocal and whole body actions. Mirror neurons (Sinigaglia, 2008) may explain the brain mechanism for theory of mind, but mother-infant interaction provides the means by which it occurs. Elders provide alternative and more intensive means to accomplish what mothers do for infants the world over. Perhaps people diagnosed with autism are less primed to engage their mothers in non-verbal dialogue, perhaps their mothers get frustrated by their lack of response, or perhaps their mothers are not appropriately shaped by the infants. Whatever the reason, we suspect that the ceremonies and practices of the elders are intensively providing some correction or rehabilitation of these pre-existing disabilities.

In each of my stories, the elders relied heavily upon drumming and singing to integrate the diagnosed with autism individuals into their circles of concern. In keeping with their general approach, they were completely permissive and non-judgmental, refusing to accept the autism diagnosis. Rather, as one elder said, "That's just how Michael is. He's ok. When he wants to be different, he will be. Until then, let him be." Within this permissive and accepting approach, Michael was encouraged to attend all ceremonies and powwows. The protection of the elder assured a minimum of teasing. Michael was encouraged to dance regardless of how clumsy he looked. "We dance," the elder said, "because that is our nature."

Michael attached to the drums and rattles. He could sit for hours making rhythm. Sometimes the elder would join him and they would answer each other. Slowly but surely, through drum and dance, these autistic children became integrated into the fabric of the community. They appeared to develop empathy and a science of mind.

The sharing of rhythm, song, and movement may have led these people diagnosed with autism, like young infants, to develop inter-subjective awareness (Braten, 1988, 1998). People diagnosed with autism are less likely to articulate narratives that are pleasing to others. Perhaps rhythm, music, and dance lead them to correct their earlier deficits through learning how to construct narratives without words (Gratier & Trevarten, 2008) that then prime the neural circuits to learn language and specifically the subtle give-and-take of social relationships.

Elders are adept at narratives without words. The sacred songs of ceremonies convey rich cultural messages through music. Ceremony itself is a narrative enactment. For example, the Lakota pipe ceremony continually re-enacts the gifting of the people with the sacred pipe (channupa) through which prayers are answered. The ceremony re-enacts the story in which wohpe (White Buffalo woman) brings a buffalo calf bone pipe and a pipestone stem to the people. When the proper procedure is followed (as she taught it), Wohpe enters the tobacco smoke and mediates between those praying and the Creator (Dakuskanskan), so that the prayers are answered (Walker, 1998). People diagnosed with autism are enrolled into the enactment of these ceremonies, entrained by the best of the drum, the musical narratives of the songs and the rhythm of the rattles. Their participation in the enactment of these stories immerses them in the socio-cultural context of the tribe with all its historicity.

In my experience, few living beings can ignore drumming and singing. I have used songs and drumming to get the attention of people diagnosed with mania, autism, even catatonic schizophrenia. I sit and sing, and eventually they show an interest.

Elders teach people diagnosed with autism to participate in their specific socio-cultural context through whole body communication.

Words can slowly catch up, but are not required – so different from conventional mainstream culture in which the words are everything.

Before discussing the parallels of indigenous healing with the contemporary worlds of art, music, and drama therapy, we wish to acknowledge the elders' perspective that the spirits are the source of this healing. We would be remiss not to mention the power of the spirits and the spiritual dimension.

Writers on creative and expressive arts therapies have begun to acknowledge the shared cultural roots of their practices (McNiff, 1992; Casson, 2004). The creative arts therapies (as they are today) and particularly the expressive arts, have been used with people with autism since the middle of the last century and the parallels with aboriginal practices are worth mentioning. The research into these ideas is considerable, but it is also intriguing to note the ways in which the approaches and goals of these therapies mirror those of the traditional healers. Music therapy, dance and movement therapy and drama therapy all use rhythm, song, metaphor and community building in their practices in ways that model indigenous healing. Perhaps for the same reasons as ceremony, young people with autism who share in rhythm, song and movement have shown increases in social awareness, meaningful play and communication (even if they show less skill and musical knowledge) (Agrotou 1998; Alvin and Warwick 1991; Nordoff and Robbins 1985, etc).

Like ceremony, music therapy involves children in community (increasing social awareness and awareness of others). Playing music with others may suit children with autism because it provides a social occasion where communication can be indirect. The intensity of a musical experience can be regulated and the rhythms are often adjusted to correspond with the mood of the day. Music-making with others encourage children to understand and negotiate boundaries between self and other, listen, keep time, take turns, engage in physical activity and use their voices in communication. Some researchers believe that music has qualities that are inherent to human cognitive processes, such as pre-verbal language preparation, social understanding and what might be considered social rhythms that underpin our abilities to understand the narratives of others, and to formulate our own narrative understandings and in particular that these qualities are nurtured especially in the relationship between mother and child. Trevarthen et al (1998). Trevarthen highlights the way that music provides a pre-linguistic context for language development. Other researchers have noted that participating in music making may increase tolerance for sensory stimulation, provide positive social experiences, foster relationships and otherwise be a gentle introduction to community (Woodward, 2004).

Lately, writers like Oliver Sachs have commented that we retain music in spite of cognitive disabilities or other neurological problems. Trevarthen describes these phenomena as a musical hierarchy or orchestration of self-regulation and self-organization that is fundamental to our meaning making structures. And because music is so integral to our being, by working "…to free the person's musical limitations, resistances and defenses, and by building on the strengths of his or her musical elements, components and structures within an improvisational relationship, we are simultaneously working towards healing the other aspects of her or his cognitive, physical, neurological and emotional being." (Brown, 1994: 18).

Most approaches to music therapy rely on spontaneous musical improvisation just as the elders did. Like the elders, music therapists talk of the rhythm of our heartbeat and the way it can be used to make contact. (Trevarthen et al (1998: 176) A music therapist often starts by noting the child's heart beat, and the tone and rhythm of any sounds or movement. The therapist then works from that rhythm into an improvisation session. The therapist uses percussion or tuned instruments, or her own voice, to respond creatively to the sounds produced by the client, and encourages the client to create his or her own musical language, using sounds, rhythms, the melody of their spoken voice, even cries and screams. The aim is to create a context of sound in which the client feels comfortable and confident to express, to experience a wider range of emotions, and to discover what it is like to be in a two-way communicating relationship. For a child with autism, the nonverbal expression of feelings and the unrestricted exploration of their emotions can allow him to find expression without the added pressure of verbalization. The 'sound and fury' is an exploration of meaning (Brown, 1994).

Drumming is a fundamental part of a music therapy session and there is considerable recent research to suggest that people who participate in hand-drumming circles report a number of physical, mental, spiritual, and emotional benefits, including: increased physical energy, relaxation, pain and stress relief, emotional release, coping with addictions, partaking of healthy traditional communal diets, learning to sing and gain confidence, positive thinking, connection to spiritual and cultural worlds, mutual support, and a sense of growth, peace and joy (Goudreau et al., 2008). People who drum together experience increased well-being, healing, empowerment, voice, strength, renewal, a sense of living "the good life" and motivation to care for self and others (Goudreau et al., 2008, p. 79).

Dance movement therapy is also used with autistic children and parallels what elders do. Dance movement therapy (DMT) works from the premise that the mind and body are inseparable, and that movement can be used to engage with emotions that feel 'unspeakable' (Hanna, 1987). Dance movement also works with rhythm, allowing people to investigate changes in their mood that arise with movement. DMT therapists encourage 'authentic movement', a system of moving that encourages improvisation based on emotions (Berrol, 1992). Again, a dance movement therapist will begin with the rhythm of the patient that day, to encourage embodied exploration, but will encourage social dances, dances that explore different rhythms and ways of moving. For a child with autism, the social engagement and the group activity may be useful (Ritter & Low, 1996). The language of the body considered in dance movement therapy echoes the concern for dancing not only as a place of inclusion and social support in the aboriginal community but as a place of learning through the body (Berrol, 1992).

Drama therapy is also used with autistic children and relates directly to what elders do. Drama includes physical exercises that emphasize embodiment, discovery of the way we present ourselves in roles and encourages a gently-paced exploration of the self in the context of others (Jones, 2007; Landy, 1996). Drama therapy with children with autism uses mirroring, a technique that encourages two people to mirror the movements of each other without words, which promotes understanding. Adding vocalization and then emotions can happen through mimicking correspondent facial and body tension. Therapists use a 'back to back' game that can be used to work with contact without using eye contact. This gives the patient some indication of the impact of his strength on another body. Emotions, as different social attitudes – can be sculpted on the other body, varying from low to high amount of physical contact and playing on the repertoire of different social attitudes (Jones, 2007; Laflamme, Mainguy & Meunier, 2009).

These expressive arts techniques contain many of the same goals and approaches as aboriginal healing.

Healing has been characterized as a community survival skill in ancient cultures (Dosamantes-Beaudry, 2001). Culture and traditional knowledge have been identified as key determinants of health for Aboriginal Canadians (Healey & Meadows, 2008). It seems clear that mental health therapy—which is inextricably related to physical, spiritual, and community health—must empower Aboriginal communities in order to impact positive individual identity and well-being (Kirmayer et al., 2003). Connection to community in the present and through knowledge of a collective historical past is a resilience factor for Aboriginal people (Kirmayer et al., 2003) with direct benefits on conditions like autism. While these relationships are endorsed by the discourse on healing within Aboriginal communities and increasingly in the academic and professional helping literature, scholarly evidence is required, in some arenas, to legitimize the avenue of traditional Aboriginal spirituality and culture for healing and fostering mental health.

Research is beginning to validate what has become intuitive for some, that cultural empowerment is positively, if not causally, related to increased mental well-being. The sharing, singing, drumming, dancing, spiritual healing, is fostering a sense of cultural continuity that can make a world of difference for autistic children, adults, and others with disabilities.

THE DARK SIDE OF CONSCIOUSNESS AND THE THERAPEUTIC RELATIONSHIP

Excerpted from an address to the Sixth Annual Alternative
Therapies Symposium and Exhibition, March 2002
By Larry Dossey M.D.

Following the publication of my 1993 book **Healing Words**: *The Power of Prayer andthe Practice of Medicine*, I received several letters from religious individuals who were profoundly upset. The views of prayer and healing set forth in my book differed from theirs, and they wanted to set me straight. Some of the letters dripped with venom. The writers denounced me as a heretic and blasphemer. They often inserted religious tracts that described the fires of hell-my fate-in lurid detail. The angriest letters were unsigned with no return address-a postal drive-by in which the perpetrator could not be traced. Most of the letters concluded in the same way. Although my views on prayer were completely erroneous, the writers granted that this was not my fault. Standing outside their religion, I simply could not avoid being deluded. Therefore, because of their love and concern for me, they would pray that I would see the light and understand prayer and healing correctly.

I am grateful to readers who take the time to write to me, and I usually answer their letters personally. So I initially responded to the critical letters by thanking the individuals for their concerns. Then one day I realized that these people weren't praying for me. They were using prayer as a method of manipulation and control. They wanted to force me, through their prayers, to abandon my personal beliefs and come over to their side. From my perspective their efforts were essentially a curse or hex.

In the past decade, the spirituality-and-health connection has become part of our national dialogue and has begun to command increasing attention in modern medicine. Approximately 80 of the nation's 125 medical schools now have courses that explore the correlations between religious and spiritual practices and health. Most people involved in this dialogue assume that spiritual pursuits are either effective or simply neutral. Others, on discovering empirical evidence for the effectiveness of intentions and prayers, have lapsed into a "gee-whiz-isn't-this-wonderful!" mindset. Almost never is it acknowledged that conscious intentions and prayer might actually cause harm-despite considerable evidence that they may do so, as we shall see.

When I initially began to investigate the role of consciousness in healing, I associated this phenomenon with love and compassion. It simply did not occur to me that intentions and prayer might have a malevolent side. But as I probed more deeply, it became obvious that I was dealing with a complementary phenomenon. Just as a magnet cannot exist without both a positive and a negative pole, the light and the shadow side of healing intentions began to come together in my mind. Eventually, the good and evil that are implicit in human intentions began to take their place alongside other great complementaries in life-male-female, life-death, night-day, and so on.

A recent Gallup poll in Life magazine explored the prayer habits of Americans. The survey found that 5 percent of us actually pray for harm for other people-and that's just the 1 in 20 who will admit it. When this figure is extrapolated to the population at large, it means that there are about 12 million people in the United States who are trying to harm other through prayer.

Like most people, I initially did not want to acknowledge a dark side of healing or prayer. Eventually, however, ignoring this negative side began to seem unethical. All conventional therapies, such as drugs and surgical procedures, have negative effects. Why should the therapy of human intentions be free of hazards? If they were completely harmless, they would be the only therapy known to humankind that is perfectly safe, and this seemed highly unlikely. And if we are ethically compelled to disclose the negative effect of drugs and surgical procedures, why shouldn't we openly discuss the danger of consciousness-based therapies?

Why do we turn away from these possibilities? This desire constitutes what depth psychologist call repressing the shadow-consigning our undesirable traits and qualities to the unconscious. But if we are to mature psychologically, we must drag these unlovely traits into the light of awareness, where their influence can be openly faced. As C.G. Jung said, a whole person is one who has both walked with God and wrestled with the devil. Just so, if our consciousness is to mature as a force in healing, we are going to have to own not only its positive side but its power to harm as well.

THE THERAPEUTIC RELATIONSHIP

Can the thoughts and intentions of health-care professionals affect their patients physically, nonlocally, at a distance? Should they be considered as factors in the therapeutic relationship that develops between a health-care professional and her client?

When I was in medical school a generation ago, this question was unthinkable. A good therapeutic relationship was considered to be mainly an intellectual affair. The physician acquired information about a patient by taking a history, doing a physical examination, and performing lab tests. Then he or she made (we hope) rational decisions about what to do for the patient, and that was that. I suggest that there is another side to the therapeutic relationship that is profoundly important-the distant, unbounded, nonlocal effects of our thoughts and intentions on those we serve. I propose, moreover, that these effects may function not only for good but for harm as well.

Managed health care hasn't helped the therapeutic relationship. The increasing demands made on health-care professionals in managed -care settings has escalated the frustration many physicians feel. If they are unable to deal with their hostile feelings toward "the system," they may project them onto their patients. The result may not be merely a cranky physician with no bedside manner; it may be one who harms his patients nonlocally through his negative thoughts and intentions.

I am aware of the prohibitions against these lines of thought. The tendency has been to psychologize the therapeutic relationship and to consider it limited to the doctor's office or exam room. But we must go further in conceptualizing how we relate to one another for three reasons. First, the thrust of human wisdom is in this direction. Virtually every traditional culture has affirmed a boundless view of human consciousness in which both positive and negative intentions operate nonlocally, remotely, beyond the reach of the senses. Second, the evidence flowing from controlled laboratory studies affirms this view, as we will see,. Third, sophisticated hypotheses are emerging from within science that are consistent with nonlocal expressions of consciousness.

BASIC QUESTIONS

Let's approach this issue by asking some basic questions:

1. Is it possible, in principle, for individuals to mentally influence, at a distance, inanimate objects?

In the prestigious journal *Foundations of Physics,* Radin and Nelson reported a meta-analysis of more than 800 studies conducted between 1959 and 1987 by 68 investigators involving attempts to mentally influence the performance of random-event generators. The researchers found the results to be "robust and repeatable." They further showed that the effect persisted with increasing refinement of the experiments, contradicting the claims of critics. Radin and Nelson stated, "Unless critics want to allege wholesale collusion among more than 60 experimenters or suggest a decades, there is no escaping the conclusion that (these) effects are indeed possible." Although these hundreds of studies do not involve actual prayer, they nevertheless deal with whether human intention can, in principle, affect the physical world at a distance.

2. Is it possible, in principle, for individuals to mentally influence, at a distance, the physiological function of a living organism?

Ten subjects tried to inhibit the growth of fungus cultures in the lagoratory through conscious intent by concentrating on them for 15 minutes from a distance of approximately 1.5 yards. The cultures were then incubated for several more hours. Of a total of 194 culture dishes, 151 showed retarded growth.

In a replication of this study, one group of subjects demonstrated the same effect (inhibiting the growth of fungal cultures) in 16 of 16 trials, while stationed from 1 to 15 miles away.

Sixty subjects not known to have such abilities were able both to impede and stimulate significantly the growth of bacterial cultures.

Sixty university volunteers were asked to alter the ability of a strain of the bacterium E. coli to use lactose. This strain normally mutates from the inability to metabolize lactose ("lactose negative") to the ability to use it ("lactose positive") at a known rate. The subjects tried to influence nine test tubes of bacterial cultures-three for increased mutation from lactose negative to lactose positive, three for decreased mutation, and three uninfluenced control tubes. The bacteria mutated in the direction desired by the subjects.

Seven subjects-two spiritual healers, one physician who was interested in and believed in spiritual healing, and four students with neither experience nor interest in healing-were asked to increase the growth of yeast in 120 test tubes "by the mental method of his choice." Another 120 test tubes were used as controls. The spiritual healers and the believing physician produced significant results (P<.001), and the indifferent students produced chance results.

3. Can such an effect influence healthy animals?

In 21 experiments conducted over several years, healers tried to awaken mice more quickly from general anesthesia. These experiments were increasingly refined. In one variation, only the image of the experimental mouse was projected on a television monitor to the healer in a distant room, who tried to mentally intervene via the image. Nineteen of the 21 studies showed highly significant results: earlier recovery from anesthesia in the mice to which positive mental intent was extended.

4. Can such an effect influence biochemical processes in humans?

Blood platelets isolated from healthy human volunteers were treated by a healer, who tried to influence the activity of the enzyme monoamine oxidase (MAO activity was measured before and after the mental intent in both healthy and disrupted cells. The overall effect was to increase the variability of MAO activity relative to untreated control samples (P< .001).

5. Can such an effect influence human tissue:

Thirty-two subjects mentally attempted to prevent the hemolysis of human red blood cells (RBCs) in test tubes containing a hypotonic saline solution, as measured by standard spectrophotometric techniques. Significant differences were found between the experimental and control tubes (P < .001).

6. Can such an effect influence healthy humans?

Scores of controlled studies have demonstrated the correlation of positive mental intent with improved physiological effect in human beings at a distance. This material has been the subject of several reviews. Among the studies' findings are the following:

In a double-blind experiment involving 393 persons admitted to a coronary care unit (CCU), intercessory prayer from a distance was offered to roughly half the subjects. Significantly fewer patients in the prayer group required intubation and mechanical ventilation ($P < .002$) or antibiotics ($P < .005$), had cardiopulmonary arrests ($P < .02$), developed pneumonia ($P < .03$), or required diuretics ($P < 005$). Subjects in the prayer group had a significantly lower "severity score" based on their hospital course following admission ($P < .01$).

In a double-blind experiment involving 990 consecutive patients who were admitted to the CCU, patients were randomized to receive either remote, intercessory prayer or no prayer. The first names of patients in the prayer group were given to a team of outside intercessors who prayed for them daily for 4 weeks. Patients were unaware that others were praying on their behalf, and the intercessors did not know and never met the patients. The medical course from hospital admission to discharge was summarized in a CCU course score derived from blinded, retrospective chart review. The prayed-for group had about a 10 percent advantage compared to the usual-care group ($P = .04$).

In a double-blind experiment involving 40 patients with advanced AIDS, subjects were randomly assigned to a distant healing (DH) group or to a control group. Both groups were treated with conventional medications, but the DH group received distant healing for 10 weeks from healers located throughout the United States. Subjects and healers never met. At 6 months, blind chart review found that DH subjects acquired significantly fewer new AIDS-defining illnesses ($P = .04$), were less ill ($P = .03$), and required significantly fewer doctor visits ($P = .01$), fewer hospitalizations ($P = .04$), and fewer days of hospitalization ($P = .04$). DH subjects also showed significantly improved mood compared with controls ($P = .02$).

In 13 experiments, the ability of 62 people to influence the physiology of 271 distant subjects was studied. These studies suggested that (1) the distant effects of mental imagery compare favorable to the magnitude of effects of one's individual thoughts, feelings, and emotions on one's own physiology; (2) the ability to use positive imagery to achieve distant effects is apparently widespread in the human population; (3) these effects can occur at distances up to 20 meters (greater distances were not tested); (4) subjects with a greater need to be influenced by positive mental intent-that is, those for whom the influence would be beneficial-seem more susceptible; (5) the distant effects of intentionality can occur without the recipient's knowledge; those participating in the studies seemed unconcerned that the effect could be used for harm, and no such harmful effects were seen; and the distant effect of mental intentionality are not invariable; subjects appear capable of preventing the effect if it is unwanted.

In a double-blind study of 53 postoperative men who had undergone hernia surgery, a treatment group who received distant healing by an experienced healer showed a significant improvement in 9 of 24 variables, including objective measures such as would appearance, lower incidence of fever during hospitalization, and a number of subjective attitudinal factors, including less pain and more confidence in their treatment when compared with control groups and with a group whose members listened to a suggestion tape.

In a randomized, controlled, double-blind study, intercessory prayer was defined as "any form of requesting God to bring about a desired end...Intercessors belonged to churches in the San Francisco Bay area. The results noted that 406 subjects improved significantly on 11 measures; the intercessors, interestingly, improved significantly on 10 measures, suggesting that intercessory prayer has benefits for both the recipient of prayer and the individual who is praying. Using "healing with love," a physician-healer was able to significantly decrease the number of human breast cancer cells in tissue culture dishes compared with controls (P < .001).

In an ongoing controlled study at the Duke University School of Medicine, patients receiving urgent cardiac catheterization and angioplasty were offered intercessory prayer by prayer groups around the world. Compared with patients treated conventionally, the prayed-for patients experienced a 50 to 100 percent reduction in side effects from these invasive cardiac procedures. The study is being expanded to several major hospitals throughout the United States.

In a triple-blind study involving 219 women undergoing in vitro fertilization and embryo transfer, intercessory prayer (IP) was offered for roughly half the women by prayer groups in North America and Australia. The IP group had a higher pregnancy rate compared with the no-IP rate (50% versus 26 % P = .001). The IP group also showed a higher implantation rate (16.3%, P < .001).

7. Can human intentions harm living organisms?

It is unethical to conduct experiments in humans in which the goal of the study is cause harm, but several experiments of this sort have been done in nonhumans.

Jean Barry, a French physician-researcher, asked 10 people to mentally try to inhibit the growth of a destructive fungus, Rhizoctonia solani, from a distance of 1.5 meters, in a controlled experiment. Growth of the "influenced" fungus in 195 petri dishes was significantly retarded in 151 dishes compared with controls. The possibility that these results could have occurred by chance was less than 1 in 1,000.

University of Tennessee researchers William H. Tedder and Melissa L. Monty replicated Barry's experiment in a controlled study using the same type of fungus. College students served as influencers from a distance of up to 15 miles.

Researcher Carroll B. Nash, of Philadelphia's St. Joseph's University, asked 60 student volunteers both to promote and inhibit the growth of E. Coli bacteria. In this controlled study, they were able to mentally influence the bacterial in both directions.

HOW GOOD IS THE EVIDENCE

In the late 1980's, the United States Congress asked Professor Jessica Utts, an internationally recognized mathematician and statistician from the University of California-Davis, to assess government-funded research in the field of parapsychology (psi). She assessed hundreds of studies in which individuals attempted to acquire or convey information nonlocally, at a distance, as in the above experiments. Utts first published her finding in the prestigious journal *Statistical Science* in 1991. Her final report was sent to congress in 1995 and was republished elsewhere. Among her conclusions:

Many anomalous phenomena, such as…the possible effect of prayer on healing, are amenable to rigorous study.

Using the standards applied to any other area of science, it is concluded that psychic functioning has been well established. The statistical results of the studies examined are far beyond what is expected by chance. Arguments that these results could be due to methodological flaws in the experiments are soundly refuted. Effects of similar magnitude…have been replicated at a number of laboratories across the world. Such consistency cannot be readily explained by claims of flaws or fraud.

The magnitude…exhibited appears to be in the range between what social scientists call a small and medium effect. That means that it is reliable enough to be replicated in properly conducted experiments, with sufficient trials, to achieve the long-run statistical results needed for replicability…It is recommended that future experiments focus on understanding how this phenomenon works and on how to make it as useful as possible.

The phenomenon has been replicated in a number of forms across laboratories and cultures…it would be wasteful of valuable resources to continue to look for proof. No one who has examined all of the data across laboratories, taken as a collective whole, has been able to suggest methodological or statistical problems to explain the ever-increasing and consistent results to date.

There is little benefit to continuing experiments designed to offer proof, since there is little more to be offered to anyone who does not accept the current collection of data.

In the field of distant healing alone, five systematic or meta-analytic reviews involving scores of studies and hundreds of patients have yielded positive findings. The evidence is compelling, in my judgment, that we can affect living organisms with our thoughts at a distance and that these effects can be either good or bad.

Critics often suggest that these data are misleading because researchers publish only their positive studies and squirrel away experiments that don't pan out-the so-called file drawer argument. If all these unpublished negative studies were taken into account, skeptics claim, they would statistically undermine all the positive ones. This argument is frivolous. In both the fields of parapsychology and distant healing, there are not enough researchers in both the fields of parapsychology and distant healing, there are not enough researchers in the entire world to produce a database this large. For example, psychologist Julie Milton, from the University of Edinburgh, analyzed all the so-called "free-response" psi studies conducted between 1964 and 1993 in which subjects were in an ordinary state of consciousness (as opposed to, say, a state of deep relaxation of hypnosis). The survey encompassed 78 experiments reported in 55 publications by 35 investigators; 1,158 subjects, most of whom were unselected volunteers, were studied. Milton discovered that the overall effects resulted in odds against chance of 10 million to 1. The effects did not differ significantly among the 35 experimenters. Milton's analysis of the file-drawer issue found that 866 unsuccessful, unpublished studies would be required to abolish the overall effect.

NURSING AND THE THERAPEUTIC RELATIONSHIP

Florence Nightingale, the founder of secular nursing, vigorously championed the the value of love, compassion, and spirituality in the therapeutic relationship between a nurse and her patient. She saw not conflict between these factors and a scientific approach to nursing. Largely as a result of her prophetic vision, the profession of nursing has been years ahead of the medical profession in recognizing the value of empathy and trust in healing as exemplified by the outstanding contributions of nurse theorists such as Martha Rogers, Jean Watson, Margaret Newman, Peggy L. Chinn, and many others. The American Holistic Nurses' Association has long championed the view that caring and compassion are crucial to the core mission of nursing. Nurses also are reclaiming the title of "healer" and the concept of "healing" terms that, oddly enough, still make many physicians uncomfortable. Physicians do not have to reinvent the wheel; we have only to explore the work done by our nursing colleagues to see what the therapeutic relationship can be like.

MEDICAL HEXES

Unless health-care professionals acknowledge the capacity of our thoughts for harm, we remain blind to the harm we cause others through our mental behaviors. Andrew Weil, MD, director of the Program in Integrative Medicine at the University of Arizona in Tucson, relates an encounter with a patient who came to see him for a second opinion. "You wouldn't believe what those doctors did to me," she said. "The head neurologist took me into his office and told me I had multiple sclerosis. He let that sink in; then he went out of the room and returned with a wheelchair. Then he told me to sit in. I said, "Why should I sit in your wheelchair?" He said I was to buy a wheelchair and sit in it for an hour a day to 'practice' for when I would be totally disabled. Can you imagine?"

Interchanges of this sort amount to medical hexing. In his book *The Lost Art of Healing,* the famous Harvard cardiologist Bernard

Lown gives several examples of "words that maim" that his patients reported from interchanges with other physicians: "you are living on borrowed time"; "Your are going downhill fast"; "The next heartbeat may be your last"; "You can have a heart attack or worse any minute"; "The...angel of death...is shadowing you"; "You are a walking time bomb"; "I'm frightened just thinking about your coronary anatomy"; "Surgery should be done immediately, preferably yesterday." To these medical hexes, Weil adds a few more: "They said there was nothing more they could do for me"; "They said I'd be dead in 6 months." Nearly everyone, it seems, has experienced this sort of medical hexing at one time or another. Consider these examples related by an editor (anonymous written communication, August 29, 2002: "You are not as well as you think you are"; "Expect the best, prepare for the worst"; "Oh, you're the one who's worse than I thought."

A classic example of how the therapeutic relationship can be manipulated for good or ill was reported by Dr. Bruno Klopfer, who was treating a man for advanced lymphoma in the 1950's. The man was terminally ill, with large tumors throughout his body and fluid in his chest. All medical therapy except oxygen had been stopped, and Klopfer believed the man would die within 2 weeks. However, in a last-ditch effort he injected Krebiozen, and experimental drug that was later said to be ineffective. Klopfer describes the amazing results:

"What a surprise was in store for me! I had left him febrile, gasping for air, completely bedridden. Now, he was, walking around the ward, chatting happily with the nurses, and spreading his message of good cheer to anyone who would listen...The tumor masses had melted like snow balls on a hot stove, and in only these few days they were half their original size! This is, of course, far more rapid regression than the most rapid regression than the most radiosensitive tumor could display under heavy x-ray given every day...And he had no other treatment outside of the single useless "shot."

Within 10 days the man was practically free of disease. He began to fly his private airplane again. His improvement lasted for 2 months, until reports cropped up denouncing Krebiozen. When he read them, the man appeared cursed, and his attitude and medical condition quickly returned to a terminal state. At this point, Klopfer urged the man to ignore the negative news reports because a "new super refined, double-strength product" was now available-a complete fabrication-and injected him with sterile water. The man's response this time was even more dramatic than initially, and he resumed his normal activities for another 2 months. But his improvement ended when the American Medical Association released a report stating that nationwide tests had proved Krebiozen worthless in the treatment of cancer. A few days after reading this statement, he was admitted to the hospital, and 2 days following admission he died.

THE POSSIBLE

When I think about what the therapeutic relationship could be like I often think of Sir William Osler (1849-1919), who is widely regarded as the most influential physician in the history of modern medicine. After revolutionizing the way medicine was taught and practiced in the United States and Canada, Osler was lured to England in 1905, when the physician was at his peak of his fame. There he became the Regius Professor of Medicine at Oxford. One day he went to graduation ceremonies, wearing his splendid academic robes. On the way he stopped by the home of his friend and colleague, Ernest Mallam. One of Mallam's young sons was sick with whooping cough and bronchitis. The child appeared to be dying, and he would not respond to the ministrations of his parents or the nurses. Osler loved children greatly and had a special way with them. He adored playing with children, and they would invariably admit him into their world. So when Osler appeared in his ceremonial robes, the little boy was captivated. Never had he seen such a thing! After a brief examination, Osler sat down at the bedside. He selected a peach from a bowl of fruit and peeled, cut and sugared it. Then he fed it bit by bit to the enthralled patient. Although Osler felt recovery was unlikely, he returned for the next 40 days, each time dressed in his robes, and personally fed the young child nourishment. Within just a few days the tide had turned and the little boy's recovery became obvious.

We are at a hellish moment in history in which raw hatred between cultures, nations, and religions is at a fever pitch. The dark side of consciousness is flexing its power and can be intimidating. This is nothing new. During the darkest days of World War II, when Britain was on its knees before the onslaught of Nazism, Churchill rallied the citizens' spirits. "If you're going through Hell, keep going," he said.

Just so, if we stop during our hellish trials, Hell wins. But if we maintain our vision and carry on, we will come through and our world will be transformed. The vision that will carry us through, however, is not one that sanitizes consciousness and denies its dark side but one that recognizes its eternal polarities.

So here's what I wish I'd said to those pesky letter writers: Do not despair that a dark side of consciousness exists, that our thoughts and prayers can harm as well as heal. Just as shadows always yield to light, illness, on some level, always gives way to the love, compassion, and deep caring that Osler brought to a dying boy's bedside. That does not mean that illness is always vanquished but rather that it is transformed through the realization that consciousness is boundless, nonlocal, and infinite, thus indestructible and immortal. Love changes the end game; tragedy and annihilation are trumped.

It's the sort of thing Osler knew in his blood and that continues to whisper in ours.

Larry Dossey, a distinguished Texas physician, is deeply rooted in the scientific world, and has become an internationally influential advocate of the role of the mind in health and the role of spirituality in healthcare. Bringing the experience of a practicing internist and the soul of a poet to the discourse, Dr. Larry Dossey offers panoramic insight into the nature and the future of medicine.

Upon graduating with honors from the University of Texas at Austin, Dr. Dossey worked as a pharmacist while earning his M.D. degree from Southwestern Medical School in Dallas, 1967. Before completing his residency in internal medicine, he served as a battalion surgeon in Vietnam, where is was decorated for valor. Dr. Dossey helped establish the Dallas Diagnostic Association, the largest group of internal medicine practitioners in that city, and was chief of Staff of Medical City Dallas Hospital in 1982.

An education steeped in traditional Western medicine did not prepare Dr. Dossey for patients who were blessed with "miracle cures," remissions that clinical medicine could not explain." Almost all physicians possess a lavish list of strange happenings unexplainable by normal science," says Dr. Dossey. "A tally of these events would demonstrate, I am convinced, that medical science not only has not had the last word, it has hardly had the first word on how the world works, especially when the mind is involved."

The author of nine books and numerous articles, Dr. Dossey is the form er Executive Editor of the peer-reviewed journal Alternative Therapies in Health and Medicine, the most widely subscribed-to journal in its field. The primary quality of all of Dr. Dossey's work is scientific legitimacy, with an insistent focus on "what the data show."

As a result, his colleagues in medical schools and hospitals all over the country trust him, honor his message, and continually invite him to share his insights with them. He has lectured all over the world, including major medical schools and hospitals in the United State-Harvard, Johns Hopkins, Cornell, the Universities of Pennsylvania, California, Washington, Texas, Florida, Minnesota, and the Mayo Clinic.

The impact of Dr. Dossey's work has been remarkable. Before his book Healing Words was published in 1993, only three U.S. medical schools had courses devoted to exploring the role of religious practice and prayer in health; currently, nearly 80 medical schools have instituted such courses, many of which utilize Dr. Dossey's works a textbooks. In his 1989 book Recovering the Soul, he introduced the concept of "nonlocal mind"-mind unconfined to the brain and body, mind spread infinitely throughout space and time. Since then, "nonlocal mind" has been adopted by many leading scientist as an emerging image of consciousness. Dr. Dossey's ever-deepening explication of nonlocal mind provides a legitimate foundation for the merging of spirit and medicine. The ramifications of such a union are radical and call for no less than the reinvention of medicine.

In 1993 Dr. Dossey served on Hillary Rodham Client's Task Force on Health Care Reform.

INFORMATION AND HELP LINKS FOR
PARENTS & DOCTORS & TEACHERS

www.klinghardtneurobiology.com
Dietrich Klinghardt MD, PhD offers Family Weekend workshops for health care practitioners, students, parents, patients and interested teenagers. The workshop is based on the Bert Hellinger's family constellation approach by mending the mother/father imprints of unresolved pain, conflict, traumatic experiences and unconscious longings, transferred to the child shortly after conception.

---

www.psychologyinfo.com
Psychology Information Online provides a central place on the internet about the practice of psychology and information about psychological diagnosis,disorders, and problems, psychotherapy, and counseling (including family therapy, couple counseling, and group therapy, behavior therapy (stress management and relaxation skills training, assertiveness training, desensitization for phobias, parenting skills, etc.) psychological evaluations and testing. We also provide information about Forensic psychology and psychological consultations for legal matters.

---

www.mentalhealth.com/mind
Discussion groups, diagnosis, mental disorders, help and research links.

---

www.addwarehouse.com
    Resource site for developmental disorders.

_____

www.autismspeaks.org
    Family services, networking, news, research, events, community.

_____

www.alternativementalhealth.com
    Mental health approaches.

_____

www.mentalhelp.net
    Information, links and referrals.

_____

www.nativeremedies.com
    An excellent website to obtain free homeopathic information about mental and behavior remedies from herbalists, naturopaths, and homeopaths. They claim to offer answers to your questions within 24 hours.

_____

www.greatplainslaboratory.com
    Online biomedical testing for toxins. Free testing information for Autism and behavior disorders.

_____

www.thingsherbal.com
    Online Alternative Medicine

_____

www.brainmattersinc.com
Information on high definition SPECT imaging of the brain for mental and behavior disorders.

---

www.healnaturally.net
Body scan information

---

www.amfundation.org
Alternative Medicine Foundation provides evidence-based research resources for consumers about alternatives to conventional western medicine.

---

www.latitudes.org
Association for Comprehensive NeuroTherapy (ACN) features a newsletter dealing with alternative treatments for Tourette Syndrome, ADD, ADHD, Autism and learning disabilities.

---

www.winhs.org
World Institute of Natural Health Sciences established to support and defend the natural and alternative health care industries.

---

www.gcnm.com
Alternative Holistic Health Study of Nutrition and Herbs.

---

www.connecticutcenterforhealth.com
Online lab testing/Natural Treatments/Free Newsletter

---

http://www.eeginfo.com
Neurofeedback/Therapeutic Applications/Tourette Syndrome/
Trauma/Temper Tantrums

_____

www.kotsanisinstitute.com
   Biomedical testing and treatments for Autism and Spectrum
   disorders

_____

www.mehl-madrona.com
Healing workshops and online courses.

_____

http://carecreditworks.com/
Credit plans for patients to use when unable to pay for treatment.

_____

www.generationrescue.org
Autism treatment information and community.

_____

www.talkaboutcuringautism.org
Information about diet, health insurance, biomedical, parent
mentoring & more.

_____

www.amfoundation.org
Information on the integration of alternative and conventional
medicine.

_____

www.verdant.net

Grow your own organic vegetables! This is not as complicated as you might think. If you have access to a deck, a roof, a patch of ground no larger than a flower bed or far more space, you can, with just a few of the resources listed on this page learn to feed yourself and others.

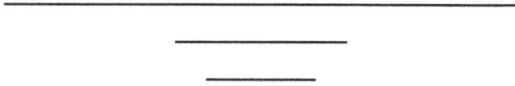

Notes and References

Indigenous Approaches To Healing
With Special Reference To Autism

Abrahamsen, V. (1997). The goddess and healing: Nursing's heritage from antiquity. *Journal of Holistic Nursing, 15*, 9-24.

Agrotou, A. (1988). A case study Lara. Journal of British music therapy. 2(1), pp. 17-23.

Allen, P. G. (1992). The sacred hoop: Recovering the feminine in American Indian traditions. Boston: Beacon Press.

Alvin, J. and Warwick, A. (1991). Music therapy for the autistic child. 2nd ed. Oxford: Oxford University Press.

Amadahy, Z. (2003). The healing power of women's voices. In K. Anderson & B. Lawrence (Eds.), *Strong women stories: Native vision and community survival* (pp. 144-155). Toronto: Sumach Press.

Anderson, K. (2000). A recognition of being: Reconstructing native womanhood. Toronto: Second Story Press.

Baird-Olson, K., & Ward, C. (2000). Recovery and resistance: The renewal of traditional spirituality among American Indian women. *American Indian Culture and Research Journal, 24*, 1-35.

Bateson MC. (1979). The epigenesist of conversational interaction: a personal account of research development. In M. Bullowa (ed.). *Before Speech: the beginning of human communication.* London: Cambridge University Press, pp. 63-77.

Bennett, M. (2005). *An annotated overview of research on Aboriginal women, health and healing.*

Vancouver: Aboriginal Women's Health and Healing Research Group. Retrieved October 14, 2008 from, http://www.awhhrg.ca/docs/annotated_bib_AWHHRG.pdf

Berrol, C. (1992) The neurophysiological basis of the mind-body comnnection in dance/movement therapy. *American journal of dance therapy 14(1).*

Braten S. (1988). Dialogic mind: the infant and adult in protoconversation. In M.E. Carvallo (ed.). *Nature, cognition, and system.* Dordrecht: Kluwer.

Braten S. (1998), Intersubjective communion and understanding: development and perturbation. In Stein Braten (ed.), *Intersubjective communication and emotion in early ontogeny.* Cambridge: Cambridge University Press, pp. 372-382.

Brown, S. M. K. (1994). Autism and music therapy: is change possible, and why music? Journal of British music therapy. 8(1), pp. 15-25.

Chandler, M. J., & Lalonde, C. E. (1998). Cultural continuity as a hedge against suicide in Canada's First Nations. *Transcultural Psychiatry, 35,* 191-219.

Chandler, M. J., & Lalonde, C. E. (2004). Transferring whose knowledge? Exchanging whose best practices?: On knowing about Indigenous knowledge and Aboriginal suicide. In J. P. White, P. Maxim, & D. Beavon (Eds.), *Aboriginal Policy Research: Setting the Agenda for Change, vol. 2.* Toronto: Thompson.

CRIAW (Canadian Research Institute for the Advancement of Women) (2008). *Aboriginal women healing themselves, their families and their communities: The case of the Minwaashin Lodge.* Retrieved October 14, 2008 from, http://www.criaw-icref.ca/Alternative%20Case %20Studies/Minwaashin_e.pdf

Crowe-Salazar, N. (2007). Exploring the experiences of an elder, a psychologist and a psychiatrist: How can traditional practices and healers complement existing practices in mental health. *First Peoples Child & Family Review, 3*, 83-95.

Dosamantes-Beaudry, I. (2001). The suppression and modern re-emergence of sacred feminine healing traditions. *The Arts in Psychotherapy, 28*, 31-37.

Finkler, K. (2004). Traditional healers in Mexico: The effectiveness of spiritual practices. In U. P. Gielen, J. M. Fish & J. G. Draguns (Eds.), *Handbook of culture, therapy, and healing* (pp. 161-174). Mahwah, NJ: Lawrence Erlbaum Associates.

Gone, J. P. (2007). "We never was happy living like a Whiteman": Mental health disparities and the postcolonial predicament in American Indian communities. *American Journal of Community Psychology, 40*, 290-300.

Goudreau, G., Weber-Pillwax, C. W., Cote-Meek, S., Madill, H., & Wilson, S. (2008). Hand drumming: Health-promoting experiences of Aboriginal women from a Northern Ontario urban community. *Journal of Aboriginal Health, 4*, 72-83.

Gratier M, Trevarthen C. (2008). Musical narrative and motives for culture in mother-infant vocal interaction. In Whitehead C. (ed.). The Origin of Consciousness in the Social World. Exeter, UK: Imprint Academica.

Hanna, J. (1987). *To dance is human: A theory of nonverbal communication.* Chicago: University of Chicago Press

Health Canada (2007). First Nations, Inuit, and Aboriginal health: Mental health and wellness. Retrieved December 12, 2008 from, http://www.hc-sc.gc.ca/fniah-spnia/promotion/mental/index-eng.php

Heilbron, C. L., & Guttman, M. A. J. (2000). Traditional healing methods with First Nations women in group counselling. *Canadian Journal of Counselling, 34*(1), 3-13.

King, T. (2003). Interview on Massey Lecture (The truth about stories: A Native narrative.). *Daybreak*. Retrieved from http://www.cbc.da/ ideas/massey/massey2003.html November 16, 2007.

Kirmayer, L., Simpson, C., & Cargo, M. (2003). Healing traditions: culture, community and mental health promotion with Canadian Aboriginal peoples. *Australasian Psychiatry, 11,* S15-S23.

Koss-Chioino, J. D. (2004). Women as healers: A "gendered" exploration in Puerto Rico and elsewhere. In U. P. Gielen, J. M. Fish & J. G. Draguns (Eds.), *Handbook of culture, therapy, and healing* (pp. 175-188). Mahwah, NJ: Lawrence Erlbaum Associates.

Laflamme, E., Mainguy, B., Meunier, A. (2009). Creative arts therapy interventions for children with Autism. Presentation Concordia University.

Landy, R. (1996). Persona and Performance: The meaning of role in drama, therapy and everyday life. London: Guilford Press.

Lawrence, B., & Anderson, K. (2003). For the betterment of our nations. In K. Anderson & B. Lawrence (Eds.), *Strong women stories: Native vision and community survival* (pp. 12-22). Toronto: Sumach Press.

Leclair, C., Nicholson, L., & Hartley, E. (2003). From the stories that women tell: The Metis Women's Circle. In K. Anderson & B. Lawrence (Eds.), *Strong women stories: Native vision and community survival* (pp. 55-69). Toronto: Sumach Press.

Lux, M. (2007). Medicine that walks: Disease, medicine, and Canadian Plains Native people. Toronto: University of Toronto Press.

McNiff, S. (1992) Art as medicine: Creating a therapy of the imagination. Boston: Shambala

Mehl-Madrona L. (1998). *Coyote Medicine: Lessons for healing from Native America.* New York: Simon & Schuster.

Mehl-Madrona L. (2003) Coyote Healing: Miracles of Native Medicine. Rochester, VT: Bear and Company.

Mehl-Madrona L (2007). Narrative Medicine: The use of history and story in the healing process. Rochester, VT: Bear and Company.

Mooney J. (1856). The Swimmer Manuscript. Washington, DC: Smithsonian Institute.

Nordoff, P. and Robbins, C. (1985). Therapy in music for handicapped children. London: Gollancz.

O'Nell, T. M. (1996). Disciplined hearts: History, identity, and depression in an American Indian community. Berkeley: University of California Press.

Reddy V. (2008). *How infants know minds.* Cambridge, MA: Harvard University Press.

Redmond, L. (1997). When the drummers were women: A spiritual history of rhythm. New York: Three Rivers Press.

Ritther, M. & Low, K. (1996). Effects of dance movement therapy: A meta-analysis. *The arts in psychotherapy. 23(3).* 249-260.

St. Pierre, M., & Long Soldier, T. (1995). Walking in the sacred manner: Healers, dreamers, and pipe carriers—medicine women of the Plains Indians. New York: Simon & Schuster.

Shepard, B., O'Neill, L., & Guenette, F. (2006). Counselling with First Nations women: Considerations of oppression and renewal.

International Journal for the Advancement of Counselling, 28, 227-240.

Sinigaglia C. (2008). Mirror Neurons: This is the Question. In Whitehead C. (ed.). The Origin of Consciousness in the Social World. Exeter, UK: Imprint Academica.

Solomon, A., & Wane, N. N. (2005). Indigenous healers and healing in a modern world. In R.

Moodley & W. West (Eds.), *Integrating traditional healing practices into counselling and psychotherapy* (pp. 52-60). Thousand Oaks, CA: Sage Publications.

Stevenson, J. (1999). The circle of healing. *Native Social Work Journal, 2,* 8-21.

Struthers, R. (2000). The lived experience of Ojibwa and Cree women healers. *Journal of Holistic Nursing, 18*, 280-295.

Struthers, R. (2003). The artistry and ability of traditional women healers. *Health Care for Women International, 24*, 340-354.

Tedlock, B. (2005). The woman in the shaman's body: Reclaiming the feminine in religion and medicine. New York: Bantam Books.

Trevarthen C. (1974). Conversations with a two-month old. New Scientist, 2 May, pp. 230-5.

Trevarthen C. (1990). Signs before Speech. In Sebeok TA & *Umiker-Sebeok J. (eds.). The Semiotic Web. New York: Mouton de Gruyter, pp. 689-755.

Trevarthen C. (1994). Infant Semiosis. In W. Noth (ed.). Origins of Semiosis: sign evolution in nature and in culture. Berlin: Mouton de Gruyter, pp. 219-52.

Waldram, J. (2004). Revenge of the Windigo: The construction of the mind and mental health of North American Aboriginal peoples. Toronto: University of Toronto Press.

Walker (1998). Lakota Rituals and Beliefs. Lincoln, NE: University of Nebraska Press.

Waldram, J. (1997). The way of the pipe: Aboriginal spirituality and symbolic healing in Canadian prisons. Peterborough, ON: Broadview Press.

1   **Case study reports in this text are from work by Dr. Mehl-Madrona. For the purposes of grammatical simplicity, we have used "I" in reference to those.
    Address communication to Dr. Lewis Mehl-Madrona, Department of Psychology, Argosy University Hawaii, 1001 Bishop St, ASB Tower, 4ᵗʰ Floor, Honolulu, HI 96813. Email is** mehlmadrona@gmail.com. **mehlmadrona.com**
2   **Within this article, we have primarily consider the indigenous cultures of North America, with which the author is most familiar, especially those of the Northern Plains.**

Notes and References
The Dark Side of Consciousness
And The Therapeutic Relationship
By Larry Dossey/Courtesy Larry Dossey
www.dosseydossey.com

NOTES

1. Richard's story is true, but I have changed his name and key events to preserve his anonymity. This applies also to all the other clinical stories in this essay.

2. The logjam of managed care may be breaking up.

3. We are in the midst of a Nightingale renaissance. In 2001 she was honored by being included in *Book of Lesser Feasts and Fasts* of the Episcopal Church of the United States, with a commemorative service in September in Washington's National Cathedral.

References

1. Dossey L: Healing Words: The power of prayer and the practice of medicine, San Francisco, 1993, Harper San Francisco

2. Levin JS: How religion influences morbidity and health: reflections on natural history, salutogenesis and host resistance, Soc Sci Med 43(5):849-854, 1996.

3. Levin J: God, faith, and health, New Yourk, 2002, John Wiley & Sons.

4. Better times for spirituality and healing in medicine, Res News Opportun Sci Theol/1 (6):12, 2001.

5. Clarke CJS. The nonlocality of mind. J Consciousness Stud. 1995; 2(3):231-40.

6. Jahn RG, Dunn BJ: A modular model of mind/matter manifestations (M5), J Sci Explor 15(3):299-329,2001.

7. Radin D: The conscious universe, San Francisco, 1997, Harper San Francisco, pp. 2788-287.

8. Rauscher EA, Targ R: The speed of thought: investigation of a complex space-time metric to describe psychic phenomena, J Sci Explor 15(3):331-354, 2001.

9. Walach H: Theory and apory in healing research: "influence" versus "correlational" models, Subtle Energ Energ Med 11(3):189-205, 2002.

10. Radin DI, Nelson RD: Evidence for consciousness-related anomalies in random physical systems, Found Physical Systems, Found Phys 19:1499-1514, 1989.

11. Barry J: General and comparative study of the psychokinetic effect on a fungus culture, J Parapsychol 32:237-243, 1968.

12. Tedder WH, Monty ML: Exploration of long-distance PK: a conceptual replication of the influence on a biological system. In Roll WG, Beloff J, Editors: Research in parapsychology 1980, Metuchen, N.J., 1981, Scarecrow Press, PP. 90–93.

13. Nash CB: Psychokinetic control of bacterial growth, J Am Soc Psychical Res 51:217-221, 1982.

14. Nash CB: Test of psychokinetic control of bacterial mutation, J Am Soc Psychical Res 78(2):145-152,1984.

15. Haraldsson E, Thorseteinsson T: Psychokinetic effects on yeast. An exploratory experiment. In Roll WG, Morris RL, Morris JD,

Editors: Research in parapsychology 1972, Metuchen, N.J., 1973, Scarecrow Press, pp. 20-21.

16. Watkins GK, Watkins AM: Possible PD influence on the resuscitation of anesthetized mice, J Parapsychol 35(4):257-272, 1971.

17. Watkins Gk, Watkins AM, Wells RA: Further studies on the resuscitation of anesthetized mice. In Roll WG, Morris RL, Morris JD, Editors: Research in parapsychology 1972, Metuchen, N.J., 1973, Scarecrow Press, pp. 157-159.

18. Wells R, Klein J: A replication of a "psychic healing" paradigm, J Parapsychol 36:144-147, 1972.

19. Wells R, Watkins G: Linger effects in several PK experiments. In Morris JD, Roll WG, Morris RL, Editors: Research in parapsychology 1974, Metuchen, N.J., 1975, Scarecrow Press, pp. 143-147.

20. Rein G: A psychokinetic effect on neurotransmitter metabolism: alterations in the degradative enzyme monoamine oxidase. In Weiner DH, Radin D, Editors: Research in parapsychology 1985, Metuchen, N.J., Scarecrow Press, pp. 77-80, 1986.

21. Braud W: Distant mental influence of rate of himolysis of human red blood cells, J Am Soc Psychical Res 84(1-24, 1990.

22. Benor DJ: Healing research, vols. 1-2, Munich, 1993, Helix Verlag.

23. Solfvin J: Mental healing. In Krippner S, Editor: Advances in parapsychological research, Jefferson, N.C., 1984, McFarland, pp.31-63.

24. Byrd Rd: Positive therapeutic effects of intercessory prayer in a coronary care unity population, South Med J 81 (7):826-829, 1988.

25. Harris W et al: A randomized, controlled trial of the effects of remote, intercessory prayer on outcomes in patients admitted to the coronary care unit, Arch Intern Med 159(19)2273-2278,1999.

26. Sicher F et al: A randomized double-blind study of the effect of distant healing in a population with advanced AIDS-report of a small-scale study, West J Med 169(6):356-363, 1998.

27. Braud W, Schlitz M: Psychokinetic influence on electrodermal activity, J Parapsychol 47(2):95-119, 1983.

28. Braud W, Schlitz M: Possible role of intuitive data sorting in electrodermal biological psychokinesis (bio-PK). In Weiner DH, Morris RL, Editiors: Research in parapsychology 1987, Me tuchen, N.J., 1988, scarecrow Press, pp. 5-9.

29. Braud W, Schlitz M: a methodology for the objective study of transpersonal imagery, J Sci Explor 3(1):43-63, 1989.

30. Bentwich Z, Kreitler S: Psychological determinants of recovery from hernia operations. Paper presented at Dead Sea Conference, June 1994, Tiberias, Israel.

31. O'Laoire S: An experimental study of the effect of distant, intercessory prayer on selfesteem, anxiety, and depression, Altern Ther Health Med 3(6):38-53, 1997.

32. Smith AL, Laskow L: Intentional healing in cultured breast cancer cells. In Proceedings of the 25th meeting of the Academy of Religion and Psychical Research, June 2000, Rosemont,Pa.

33. Krucoff M: The Mantra study project [interview], Altern Ther Health Med 5(3): 74-82, 1999.

34. Krucoff MW al: Integrative noetic therapies as adjuncts to percutaneous intervention during unstable coronary syndromes:

Monitioring and Actualization of Noetic Training (MANTRA) feasibility pilor, Am Heart J 142(5): 760-767, 2001.

35. Utts J: Replication and meta-analysis in parapsychology, Statist Sci 6: 363-403, 1991.

36. Utts J: An assessment of the evidence for psychic functioning, J Parapsychol 59:289-320, 1995

37. Utts J: An assessment of the evidence for psychic functioning, J Sci Explor 10(1):3-30, 1996.

38. Utts J: The significance of statistics in mind-matter research, J Sci Explor 13(4):615-638, 1999.

39. Astin JA, Harkness E, Ernst E: The efficacy of "distant healing" a systematic review of randomized trials, Ann Intern Med 132:903-910, 2000.

40. Abbot NC: Healing as a therapy for human disease: a systematic review, J Altern complement Med 6(2):159-169, 2000.

41. Braud W. Schlitz M: A methodology for the objective study of transpersonal imagery, J Sci Explor 3(1):43-63, 1989.

42. Jonas WB: The middle way: realistic randomized controlled trials for the evaluation of spiritual healing, J Altern Complement Med 7(1):5-7, 2001.

43. Schiltz M, Braud W: Distant intentionality and healing: assessing the evidence, Altern Ther Health Med 3(6):62-73, 1997.

44. Milton J: Ordinary state ESP meta-analysis. In Schlitz MF, Editor: Proceedings of the36th annual meeting of the Parapsychological Association, August 1993, Toronto, Ontario.

45. Dossey BM: Florence Nightingale: mystic, visionary, healer, Springhouse, Pa, 2000, Stringhouse.

46. Paris MR: Letter to the editor, JAMA 287,2002.

47. Marriner-Tomey A: Nursing theorists and their work, ed 3, St. Louis, 1994, Mosby.

48. Rogers ME: Nursing: a science of unitary human beings. In Riehl-Sisca J, Editor: Conceptual models for nursing practice, ed 3 Norwalk, Conn, 1989, Appleton & Lange.

49. Watson J: Nursing: human science and human care, Norwalk, Conn, 1985, Appleton Century-Crofts.

50. Newman MA: Newman's health theory. In Clements IW, Roberts FB, Editors: Family health: a theoretical approach to nursing care, New York, 1983, John Wiley & Sons.

51. Chinn PL: Theory and nursing, ed 5, St. Louis 1999, Mosby.

52. Dossey BM, Keegan L, Guzzetta CE: Holistic nursing: a handbook for practice, ed 3, Gaithersburg, Md, 2000, Aspen.

53. Frisch NC et al: AHNA standards of holistic nursing proctice, guidelings for caring and healing, Gaithersburg, MD 2000, Aspen.

54. Keegan L, Dossey BM: Profiles of nurse healers, New York, 1998, Delmar.

55. Weil A: spontaneous healing, New York, 1995, Alfred A. Knopf, pp. 63-64.

56. Lown B: The Lost Art of Healing, New Yourk, 1996, Hourghton-Mifflin, p. 65.

57. Klopfer B: Psychological variables in human cancer, J Proj Tech 21: 331-340, 1957.

58. Golden RL: William Osler at 150. An overview of a life, JAMA 282(23):2252-2258, 1999.

59. Robinson JC: The end of managed care, JAMA 285(20):262202628, 2001.

BOOKS BY CONTRIBUTING AUTHORS OF
FATAL WORDS FRAGILE HOPES

LARRY DOSSEY, MD

**The Power of Premonitions
The Extra-Ordinary Healing
(The Power of Ordinary Things)
Healing Beyond The Body
Reinventing Medicine
Be Careful What You Pray For
Prayer Is Good Medicine
Healing Words
Meaning and Medicine
Recovering The Soul
Space Time and Medicine**

LEWIS MEHL-MADRONA, MD, Ph.D, Mphil

**Healing The Mind Through The Power of Story
(The Promise of Narrative Psychiatry)
Narrative Medicine
Coyote Wisdom
Coyote Healing**

SEAON DUCOTE

**The Illusion of Age/Fallacy of Decline
The Illusion of Age/Fallacy of Time
Fatal Words Fragile Hopes
In Our Image
Remnants**

www.ingramcontent.com/pod-product-compliance
Lightning Source LLC
Chambersburg PA
CBHW020612270326
41927CB00005B/294